GLP-1 Weight Loss Blueprint

The Breakthrough Approach to Reduce Cravings, Eat Healthy, and Make This the Last Diet You'll Ever Need

Lauren Pierce

Revised Edition 2026

ISBN 978-1-0697304-3-5

CONTENTS

Introduction

I never planned on becoming an expert in chronic pain or weight loss. Twenty-five years ago, when a back injury upended my life as a teenager, I was told to rest, heal, and eventually move on. Instead, I entered a decades-long maze of multiple surgeries, physical therapy sessions in sterile rooms, every diet with a promise (keto, paleo, intermittent fasting), and every supplement that claimed to be the answer.

But the longer I searched for answers, the more complex things became. The pain was relentless, but it wasn't just about hurting. It was the exhaustion of living in constant fight-or-flight mode, watching my weight refuse to budge no matter what I tried, feeling like my body had locked me out of my own life.

If you are reading this book, you probably know exactly what I mean. Maybe you've spent late nights diving into the latest health breakthroughs, scrolling through Reddit threads and Instagram hashtags, tracking your steps and glucose levels with apps and wearables, all while juggling work deadlines and family chaos. Perhaps you've paid for premium insurance plans, tried countless online fitness programs, ordered organic groceries, and even hired health coaches, all in search of more energy, better mobility, and greater control over your future.

And yet here we are. Cravings still hit at 9 p.m. The scale seems immune to your best efforts. Every bite is a calculation, every workout measured against a metabolism that feels broken. And perhaps the hardest part isn't always the physical struggle, it's the emotional exhaustion of hope, effort, disappointment, and repeat. You're not broken, and you're definitely not failing. For educated, resourceful, and informed people entering their forties, fifties, and beyond, the path to sustainable weight loss feels rigged against us.

Especially if you're also dealing with type 2 diabetes, prediabetes, PCOS, thyroid issues, insulin resistance, or any of the other metabolic curveballs that life throws right when everything else is demanding your attention. This book exists because I am one of you, and I know what it means to want more than another quick fix.

I learned the hard way that real solutions are buried under mountains of hype, miracle diets that work for two weeks, and empty promises. Social media is full of before-and-after photos and influencers selling detox teas, and experts hawking secrets they've trademarked. You've probably tried enough of these so-called answers to fill a medicine cabinet. But beneath all that noise lives a real, evidence-backed breakthrough: GLP-1 therapies.

GLP-1 is short for glucagon-like peptide-1 receptor agonists. It is changing the conversation about obesity, hunger, blood sugar, and how our bodies process food. These aren't supplements or another fad; they represent a breakthrough that leading institutions like the Mayo Clinic, American Diabetes Association (ADA), and researchers publishing in the New England Journal of Medicine describe as "paradigm-shifting." Originally developed to treat type 2 diabetes, GLP-1s, such as Ozempic and Wegovy, work by targeting how hormones regulate hunger, fullness, blood sugar, and fat storage (Adkison, 2022). Clinical trials into GLP-1s demonstrate sustained weight loss and metabolic improvements that traditional diet and exercise alone rarely deliver, especially for those of us who have followed the rules for years without seeing results (Schnabel, 2025).

Let me be clear upfront: This isn't magic. No injection, pill, smoothie, or app will transform your life overnight. Sustainable weight loss, especially after forty, involves more than what you eat or don't eat. It's about understanding the biology behind cravings, hormonal shifts, gut health, sleep, stress, and, yes, the modern medications that can finally unstick what's been stuck for years. That's exactly what this book delivers: a blueprint rooted in real research, clinical evidence, and personal experience. This is not another unsustainable fad.

So what makes this different from everything else you've read? First, I've lived it. The back surgery that failed. The years on painkillers. The weight that crept on despite doing everything "right."

The moment I finally found something that worked. Second, everything here is designed for your actual life: packed calendars, skepticism earned through experience, and zero patience for fluff. Each chapter provides practical strategies for busy routines and honest conversations about obstacles, from navigating insurance companies and managing side effects to finding nutrition and fitness habits that work in the real world, not on someone else's Instagram highlight reel.

Inside, we'll break down the building blocks of GLP-1 therapy: How these medications work in your body, why they succeed where intermittent fasting or restrictive diets fail for many of us, which side effects actually matter and how to handle them, how to get your insurer on board (or plan for out-of-pocket costs), and, most importantly, how to stay motivated when progress ebbs and flows.

Skeptical? I hope so. In fact, I encourage it. As a lifelong student of both science and self-experimentation, I believe you should question every claim, including mine. That's why every recommendation is supported by references from peer-reviewed studies, guidelines from respected medical organizations, and real clinical trial data. If you're a data-driven thinker who's used to cross-referencing Healthline, PubMed, or Peter Attia's podcasts, you'll find citations and research notes throughout, so you never have to take my word for it.

But data alone won't change anything. That's where this book goes beyond theory. You'll find step-by-step guides on how to approach your doctor, what questions will get you answers, sample scripts for discussing GLP-1s with your care team, day-one checklists, and tracking tools to monitor progress and troubleshoot problems. We'll talk honestly about the stuff nobody mentions: the guilt of needing medical help instead of relying on "willpower," the sometimes awkward conversations about injections or cost, the reality of plateaus, and the voice in your head that whispers you're not doing enough.

Practical tips are tailored for people trying to cook healthier meals between Zoom calls, fit micro-workouts around travel, or balance wellness goals with caregiving responsibilities. Just as important, this book connects you to others walking the same path, a growing network of GLP-1 users who share meal ideas, troubleshoot insurance denials, trade nausea remedies, celebrate wins, and remind each other that progress doesn't have to be perfect to be real. Let me also be upfront about what this book won't do. It won't promise miracles, guarantee overnight success, or pretend side effects are no big deal. This isn't an advertisement for a single brand or medical practice. Instead, this is an invitation to change that's actually sustainable, grounded in self-knowledge, modern science, and the belief that you deserve to feel at home in your body.

Here's what's coming up in the pages ahead: First, we'll dig into the science behind GLP-1s, learning why hormones and gut peptides play such a huge role in hunger and metabolism. Then, you'll get a hands-on guide for starting therapy, getting prescriptions, and managing side effects (from mild headaches to more serious concerns). The nutrition and movement chapters translate the latest research into meal plans and activity suggestions that work with your medication, not against it. Throughout, I'll share strategies for staying in the game, setting meaningful milestones, using technology for feedback, building resilience during tough stretches, and connecting with people who understand.

We'll tackle the barriers head-on, the insurance denials, judgment from others, and physician misunderstandings. And we'll give you the tools to push through anyway. Plus, reflective exercises to help you personalize your plan, document progress, and celebrate victories beyond the scale, such as reduced joint pain, clothes that fit, lower A1C, and renewed energy to actually enjoy your life, whatever that looks like.

Transformation isn't easy, but with the right knowledge, support, and tools, it is absolutely possible. I wrote this book as a companion for every person who's ever felt stuck, who wants evidence-based answers, real progress, and a community that celebrates every victory. Together, we can break the cycle of frustration and move toward real, lasting change.

You only need to take the first step. Let's get started.

Chapter 1:

From Diet Fatigue to Lasting Change: The GLP-1 Breakthrough

I've lived with pain for more than twenty-five years. A back injury in my late teens started a cycle I couldn't escape: multiple surgeries, every therapy imaginable (even stem cells), every diet trend, and every supplement that promised relief.

Yet the biggest battle wasn't just the pain itself, but what came with it: weight that refused to move, a metabolism that felt broken, and a body stuck in "fight-or-flight" mode almost all the time. Cortisol stayed elevated, my gut never fully healed, and every effort to "fix" myself seemed to hit the same invisible wall.

After my failed back surgery in 2005, I started asking different questions. Was my slowing metabolism really just a result of aging, or was it the constant stress that was flooding my system with chemicals? Were gut issues making it impossible to calm my cortisol and reset my body? And if I could reduce inflammation, would that change everything?

These questions led me down a rabbit hole of research about chronic pain, inflammation, and weight. What I discovered changed everything: the connections between these systems run deeper than I'd ever imagined, and traditional approaches to weight loss completely ignore them. Suddenly, my weight-loss journey wasn't about the scale anymore, but about giving my body a chance to heal.

This book is that journey. It's not another fad diet or empty promise. It's about understanding how pain, stress, hormones, gut health, and weight are all interconnected, and how GLP-1 therapies can help reset that cycle so lasting change is finally possible.

In this chapter, we'll explore why traditional diets often fall short and what that means for women seeking lasting change, even through the complexities of metabolism, hormones, and daily life.

The Emotional Toll of Diet Fatigue

If you've been fighting your weight for years, you know this cycle by heart. There's a familiar rhythm: a burst of hope when you find a new plan, the early weeks when everything clicks, the inevitable unraveling when cravings return, energy crashes, and then the scale creeps back.

This cycle is quietly heartbreaking for so many women, whether they are in their 30s, 40s, 50s, or beyond. Every setback whispers that maybe you're the problem, that you lack discipline or willpower. But I've learned that this isn't personal failure. Your biology is working against you.

Think back to the classic promise splashed across social media: "Drop two sizes in 30 days!" You sign up, clear out the pantry, download the tracking app, and power through awkward lunch meetings with precisely measured salads. For a few weeks, it all goes according to plan. Friends notice. The scale moves. Your inner voice dares to believe that maybe this time will be different.

Then life happens. Work gets busy, family drama explodes, or old cravings roar back to life. The plan that once seemed manageable is starting to feel rigid and joyless. You find yourself standing in the kitchen late at night, halfway through a snack you swore off, bargaining with the fridge. The weight begins to return, sometimes faster than it left, and each morning the scale seems to undo all your hard work.

The Hidden Cost of Repeated Failure

The toll goes beyond the physical. After a setback, your inner dialogue becomes harsh. *What's wrong with me? Am I broken?* The problem starts to feel like a reflection of your very character.

Many women describe keeping a mental tally of failed attempts. Some joke about their "hall of fame" of diet books; others confide that they've lost count of the number of apps they've tried.

Layla, a 48-year-old marketing director, describes her cycle perfectly: "I've probably spent over $1,000,000 over the years on programs, supplements, and gym memberships. I'd lose 30 pounds, feel amazing, then life would happen, and I'd gain back 35. Each time felt like proof that I was fundamentally broken."

Diane, a working mother of three, adds: "I used to joke that I was a professional dieter. I knew the carb counts for everything, could meal-prep like a chef, and had the discipline to follow any plan for a while. But my body seemed to have other plans. After the fifth major regain, I stopped believing change was possible."

For every regained pound, there's a heavier emotional burden. After enough cycles, even hope feels risky. What if this next attempt fails, too? The skepticism that builds doesn't come from a place of cynicism, but rather from self-protection, earned through hard experience.

That cycle of short spikes of progress, followed by long spells of disappointment, is the pattern begging for real answers. If you've wondered why, despite all your best efforts, the same frustrations return, you're not alone. There's a different set of questions to ask, and a science to explore that starts to untangle the reasons traditional approaches fail.

Why Traditional Diet Advice Falls Short

The advice is drummed into us from every angle: physicians, wellness influencers, and advertisements hawking everything from shakes to supplements. It's deceptively simple: "Eat less, move more." Got it. The problem is that this approach overlooks how the human body is designed to fight against weight loss. This oversimplification is rooted in diet culture, a system of beliefs that equates thinness with health and moral virtue while promoting weight loss at any cost.

Diet culture teaches us that if we fail to lose weight or keep it off, it's a personal moral failing rather than a predictable biological response. This blame-focused approach ignores decades of research showing that intentional weight loss fails for the vast majority of people, not because they lack character, but because they're fighting against powerful evolutionary mechanisms.

The Biology of Metabolic Resistance

When you cut calories hard, your body responds exactly as it evolved to survive: It burns fewer calories, pumps out hunger hormones, and tries to store energy at every opportunity. Reducing your intake triggers a biological alarm bell, prompting your metabolism to slow down and your appetite to rise, making it even harder to keep losing weight or maintain the loss (Tahreem et al., 2022).

Over time, each round of dieting teaches your body to be more efficient at holding on to weight. While wearing down your resolve, losing weight, especially through restriction and deprivation, actually encourages your biology to resist future attempts even more. Research consistently shows that most of the weight lost during a tightly controlled diet returns within two to five years, with as much as 80% of it regained (Hall & Kahan, 2018).

The cycle is emotionally crushing, especially when each failed attempt leaves you more doubtful about your ability to ever reach or maintain a healthy weight. It feels like running on a treadmill that speeds up every time you slow down, or carrying a backpack that gets heavier with every lap. And this is exactly how chronic dieting leaves its mark.

The Midlife Factor

For women learning how to deal with perimenopause, busy careers, caregiving responsibilities, and digital overload, the challenge becomes even more complex. The old rules rarely work and can even cause even more harm. Restrictive dieting lowers metabolic rate, disrupts hunger signals, and chips away at the motivation to keep going. (Tahreem et al., 2022).

Diet fatigue runs deeper with every failed attempt, leaving behind frustration, low motivation, and a nagging suspicion that something is amiss. But it isn't. The system is working against you.

The Breakthrough of GLP-1s

After cycling through every major diet, app, and supplement on the market, GLP-1 medications might sound like just another trend. However, the science backing these prescription medications comes straight from respected endocrinology research and medical organizations, not late-night infomercials or social media hype. Instead of targeting the surface-level effects of weight loss, GLP-1 therapies act directly in the conversation between your gut and brain, completely changing how your body manages hunger and food reward.

What Makes GLP-1s Different

GLP-1 stands for glucagon-like peptide-1. It's a hormone made naturally in your small intestine and brain. Every time you eat, GLP-1 is released into the bloodstream, helping regulate how full you feel, how quickly your stomach empties, and how your body manages blood sugar.

Today's breakthrough GLP-1 medications, such as semaglutide, liraglutide, or tirzepatide, are engineered to mimic or boost this hormone, but in ways that last longer and have a steadier, targeted effect (Amorim et al., 2025; Dailey & Moran, 2013). These aren't extracts from exotic plants or "metabolism boosters" with questionable ingredients. Each option is prescription-based and studied in thousands of people over months and years.

The main difference is that these medications tackle the drivers of weight gain and cravings at their roots. Instead of simply telling you to "eat less," they address the deeper neurobiology that makes it nearly impossible to eat less. GLP-1 signals travel to the brain, reaching sites such as the hypothalamus, the ventral tegmental area (VTA), and the nucleus accumbens. These are the regions that decide what's rewarding, when you feel satisfied, and how intense cravings become (Amorim et al., 2025). When GLP-1 binds to its receptors, neurons in these circuits start sending messages of fullness, satiety, and lowered desire for food, even when you face tempting situations that would normally trigger overeating or binge urges.

Then there's the effect on the gut. GLP-1 slows the emptying of food from your stomach into the intestine. That simple delay helps you feel full longer and steadies the spikes and drops of blood sugar that can cause intense hunger shortly after meals (Dailey & Moran, 2013). For many, this means that eating a reasonable portion finally lines up with sustained fullness and stable energy, rather than hours of white-knuckling or grazing through the afternoon. These changes can be measured. People using tools like continuous glucose monitors report visible improvements in glucose control and even describe a flattening of the usual "rollercoaster" after high-carbohydrate meals. When their medication is working, those dramatic post-meal swings become gentler curves, reflecting better hormonal tuning.

The thing that most surprised me about GLP-1 medications is that they naturally reinforce healthy eating habits in ways that go beyond appetite suppression. When I tried to eat greasy foods like burgers and fries, which I used to crave regularly, I noticed they would actually increase my discomfort and sometimes flare up my back pain. This wasn't punishment; it was my body giving me clear feedback about what worked and what didn't. The medication's side effects naturally steered me toward cleaner, more nutritious foods that felt better in my system. In many ways, this biological feedback loop became one of the most valuable aspects of the treatment, making healthy choices feel obvious rather than restrictive.

Clinical Evidence That Matters

What really sets GLP-1 therapies apart is the level of clinical validation. Large studies published in leading medical journals have tracked not only pounds lost, but changes in blood sugar, cholesterol, cardiovascular health, and patients' own ratings of food-related control (Amorim et al., 2025). These are not small, boutique studies, but the kind of evidence that causes major medical groups to update their guidelines and make these medications a new frontline option for people living with obesity or metabolic disease.

The American Diabetes Association (2024) now includes GLP-1 receptor agonists in their clinical practice guidelines for obesity management, while the Mayo Clinic describes them as game-changing medications for people who haven't succeeded with lifestyle changes alone (*Considering GLP-1 Medications?*, 2023). Compare this institutional backing to weight-loss supplements: most popular pills and powders show no measurable effect in real-world clinical trials, are not regulated for effectiveness, and are never endorsed by leading health authorities like the ADA or major medical centers.

For many people, one of the most meaningful aspects is the psychological relief that comes from finally understanding this process. GLP-1 therapies do not make you unable to enjoy food or require you to "retrain" every thought. Instead, they work by "turning down the volume" of food noise in the brain (the constant thoughts and cravings) so daily decisions feel noticeably easier and steadier, which is more than enough to shift what had been a losing battle until now (Conley, 2025).

After so many cycles of hope and disappointment, it's natural to wonder whether this is finally the answer or just another passing trend. A healthy skepticism is part of the process. The evidence and experience with GLP-1s offer something different, but every genuine breakthrough deserves a closer look, a handful of questions, and a willingness to ask, "What's the catch?"

My Personal Turning Point

For me, the change was about so much more than the weight loss. Within three months on Ozempic, I'd lost 20 pounds. But more importantly, my chronic back pain decreased significantly. Research shows that every pound of body weight lost relieves roughly four pounds of pressure on your knees, and this effect extends to other joints as well (Messier et al., 2005). Even modest weight loss doesn't just ease pressure; it reduces inflammation and can dramatically improve pain and function. I was living proof of this connection between weight and pain relief.

The real transformation was psychological. For the first time in decades, I wasn't constantly thinking about food. The 9 p.m. ice cream cravings that had sabotaged countless diets simply disappeared. I could walk past the kitchen after dinner without that magnetic pull toward the refrigerator.

This was no longer about willpower or discipline, but my biology finally working with me instead of against me. The inflammation that had been my constant companion for twenty-five years began to calm down. My sleep improved. My energy stabilized.

Most importantly, I stopped feeling like I was at war with my own body.

Beyond Weight Loss: What Real Success Looks Like

The most powerful changes often have nothing to do with the scale. People describe breakthrough moments like going an entire week without thinking about their next meal, being present at family events instead of planning what to eat afterward, or sleeping through the night without waking up hungry.

Change with GLP-1s most often starts small. Consider the story of Michelle, a 51-year-old project manager who balances work travel with menopause symptoms. Michelle describes how, week by week, she realized she was thinking about food less. She found herself able to pack her children's lunches without unconsciously nibbling on them. "I remember the day I went through a whole morning meeting and realized my stomach hadn't distracted me once." For Michelle, this wasn't an overnight transformation, but the shift felt real. The friction in her daily routine lessened, and she gained energy for things that deeply mattered to her: the time spent walking her dog after dinner or planning a vacation without secretly dreading airplane seats. Better sleep, reduced joint pain, stable energy, improved mood: these non-scale victories often matter more than pounds lost. They represent your body returning to a more natural, less stressed state.

Real success looks like eating until satisfied and naturally stopping, going hours between meals without food thoughts, making decisions about eating without internal battles, and having energy for activities you've been avoiding.

A Different Kind of Hope

I understand the skepticism. After years of disappointment, hope feels risky. What if this is just another dead end? The difference with GLP-1s is that hope isn't required upfront. You don't need to believe it will work; you just need to try it and observe what happens. The medication does the heavy lifting while you witness the changes.

This book isn't asking you to have faith in another miracle cure. Instead, it invites you to consider a scientifically backed tool that works with your biology rather than against it, and to explore whether the cycle of diet fatigue can finally be broken.

The evidence is clear. The tools are available. The question is: Are you ready to try something genuinely different?

What's Coming Next

The following chapters will give you everything you need to determine whether GLP-1 therapy is right for you and, if so, how to get started successfully. We'll cover the science behind why these medications work when diets fail, how to navigate insurance approval, what to expect in your first 90 days, and how to build sustainable habits that support long-term success.

Most importantly, we'll address the practical realities of midlife: how to fit this into a packed schedule, handle social situations, and maintain motivation when progress feels slow.

I'm going to help you find a sustainable path forward that honors both the science of weight loss and the reality of your daily life.

You've tried willpower. You've tried restriction. You've tried every trend that promised to be different. Maybe it's time to try working with your biology instead of against it.

Chapter 2:

It's Not Your Fault: The Biology of Weight and Hunger

Ever since my failed back surgery in 2005, weight has been a shadow I couldn't escape. When you can't move much, when every step feels like fire down your spine, and when the only way doctors know how to help is to hand you a prescription for T3s or morphine, the pounds start to creep on.

At first, I told myself I was just being lazy, that if I had more discipline, I'd be able to fight through it. However, living in pain isn't a sign of laziness. Living on painkillers isn't weakness.

Still, I carried the blame.

For years, I believed it was my fault. Every diet I failed. Every time the weight came back. Every look in the mirror reminded me of the person I used to be before pain changed everything. It wasn't until I started digging into the biology that I realized I'd been blaming the wrong person.

I learned about set-point theory, stress hormones like cortisol, and how the body fights to maintain weight. I realized that my body wasn't broken; it was just doing what bodies do under constant stress and pain.

In this chapter, I will help you unravel this cycle of blame and unpack the biology of weight and hunger so you can really understand what's going on beneath the surface.

The Myth of Willpower

"Why can't I just stick to it this time?" This question echoes through countless conversations between frustrated dieters and their friends, family members, and even healthcare providers. Maybe you've stared at the scale after another week of meticulous tracking that barely moved the needle. You logged every bite, walked daily, cut back on sugar, but the weight clung stubbornly, as if your efforts were invisible.

If you've ever felt this way, you're experiencing something that has nothing to do with character flaws or lack of motivation. The problem isn't that you're not trying hard enough, it's that you're fighting against biology with willpower alone.

For decades, the message has been simple: eat less, move more, try harder. If you regain weight, it likely means you got lazy or lost focus. This narrative places the entire burden on individual discipline, ignoring what science has taught us about how the body actually works. The truth is far more complex and, ultimately, far more forgiving.

When Biology Overpowers Willpower

Research shows that most diets are ineffective in the long run for the majority of people. Large studies that track people over years find that most of the weight lost is regained within one to five years (Hall & Kahan, 2018). A study from the National Institutes of Health found that for every two pounds participants lost, they consumed about 100 more calories on average during "maintenance," driven by changes in hunger hormones rather than choices (Borja, 2020). Greater restriction may even cause more intense cravings and mental fatigue, making it almost impossible for anyone to stick with cutbacks forever.

When someone loses weight through discipline and strict tracking, their body perceives a threat. Humans evolved in environments where losing fat increased the risk of starvation. Our biology responds to weight loss with a cascade of reactions designed to pull us back to where we started. Hormones shift so that ghrelin, which is known as the "hunger hormone," climbs, while leptin, which signals fullness, drops.

The brain receives signals that food is scarce, dialing up cravings and energy conservation. Muscles may burn fewer calories during rest, and the urge to eat becomes hard to ignore. It's not stubbornness or weakness. It's a survival system that works against plans and promises deeply ingrained into our physiology.

Even those who feel motivated, disciplined, and "healthy" can't outsmart these built-in responses for long. Willpower works like a muscle; it's strongest when you're rested and unstressed, but it fatigues quickly under pressure. Think about your last diet attempt. You probably started strong, full of determination and clear goals. Maybe you meal-prepped on Sundays, tracked every calorie, and felt proud of your discipline.

Then life happened. A work deadline, a family crisis, a string of bad sleep, or just the accumulating fatigue of constant restriction. Suddenly, the habits that felt manageable became overwhelming. The apple you packed for an afternoon snack got forgotten while you grabbed a candy bar from the vending machine. One slip became two, then a full return to old patterns.

Willpower is strongest in short bursts: a tough week in June, a spring diet challenge with friends. But willpower fades under stress, chronic pain, insomnia, or hormonal changes, realities that quickly stack up.

The body's feedback loops grow louder over time until a person gives in, often with shame. Dr. Angela Fitch explains, "Physiologically, as humans, we are not created to lose weight" (Borja, 2020). She points out that after rapid weight loss, our internal chemistry resets, making an individual feel hungrier and hungrier. Even high performers with old habits of persistence can't overcome hardwired signals.

More than just personal anecdotes or forum complaints, these patterns are baked into human biology. The belief that enough discipline will overpower these drives does a disservice to anyone trying to be well in a world of processed food, chronic stress, and hormonal flux. The cycle of restriction and regain reflects more about body systems than personal strength or intelligence (American Psychological Association, 2012).

Your Body's Weight Defense System

Understanding why diets fail requires understanding set-point theory. This concept suggests that your body defends a particular weight range, much like it maintains a steady body temperature. Just as you automatically shiver when cold or sweat when hot, your body has internal mechanisms that resist weight loss and push you back toward your established set point.

The Hypothalamus: Your Weight Thermostat

Deep within your brain, the hypothalamus acts as mission control for weight regulation. It receives constant updates from hormones throughout your body about energy stores, recent food intake, and stress levels. When weight drops below your set point, the hypothalamus initiates a complex response designed to restore the weight it considers "normal" (Keesey & Hirvonen, 1997).

This system evolved in response to the real threat of food scarcity. Our ancestors needed biological mechanisms to prevent dangerous weight loss during famines. Today, that same system interprets intentional dieting as a potential emergency, triggering powerful responses to restore lost weight.

Metabolic Adaptation: Your Body's Efficiency Mode

When you restrict calories, your metabolism slows down and becomes remarkably efficient. Studies of contestants from "The Biggest Loser" show that six years after dramatic weight loss, their metabolisms remained suppressed, burning 500–800 fewer calories per day than expected for their body size (Fothergill et al., 2016).

This metabolic adaptation happens to everyone who loses weight, not just reality TV contestants. Your body begins conserving energy by reducing the calories burned through daily activities, making you feel colder, more tired, and less likely to fidget or move spontaneously. Even if you maintain the same exercise routine, you're burning fewer calories than before.

The Hormone Hurricane

Weight loss triggers a cascade of hormonal changes that make regaining weight almost inevitable without ongoing intervention. Rather than being subtle shifts, these are dramatic, measurable changes that persist long after your diet ends.

Ghrelin: The Hunger Amplifier

Ghrelin, known as the hunger hormone, spikes dramatically after weight loss (Mawer, 2023). This hormone is produced in the stomach and travels to the brain, where it stimulates appetite and food-seeking behavior. After losing weight, ghrelin levels can remain elevated for a year or more, making you feel hungrier than you did before dieting.

The increase isn't modest. Studies show ghrelin can rise by 20–25% after significant weight loss (Hansen et al., 2002). This means the physical sensation of hunger becomes more intense and persistent, making it incredibly difficult to maintain new eating habits solely through willpower.

Leptin: The Missing Fullness Signal

Leptin works as the counterbalance to ghrelin, signaling fullness and telling your brain when you've had enough to eat. It's produced by fat cells, so when you lose fat, leptin levels plummet. Lower leptin means your brain receives weaker "stop eating" signals, even after a full meal (*Leptin: What It Is*, 2022).

This creates a cruel double bind: you feel hungrier due to high ghrelin levels, yet less satisfied after eating due to low leptin levels. Meals that once left you comfortably full now leave you still hungry. Hadley, a 48-year-old marketing executive, experienced this hormonal disruption firsthand after losing 35 pounds through careful calorie counting. "I remember eating a grilled chicken salad with all the vegetables and healthy fats I was supposed to have, and 30 minutes later,

I was standing in front of the refrigerator again.

My brain kept telling me I hadn't eaten enough, even though logically I knew I had. I'd lie awake at night thinking about food, planning my next meal while I was still digesting the last one. It felt like my body had forgotten how to recognize that I was fed." She later learned that this constant food preoccupation wasn't willpower failure; it was her hormones desperately trying to restore her previous weight.

Insulin: The Storage Signal

Insulin resistance often develops or worsens during cycles of weight loss and regain. When your cells become less responsive to insulin, your body compensates by producing more. Higher insulin levels promote fat storage and can trigger cravings when blood sugar drops (Chappell, 2025).

This is particularly challenging for women going through perimenopause or managing chronic stress, as both conditions can worsen insulin resistance. The result is a metabolism increasingly primed to store fat rather than burn it.

Enter GLP-1: A Different Approach

While traditional dieting fights against these biological forces, GLP-1 receptor agonists work with them. GLP-1 is a hormone naturally produced in your intestines after eating. It sends signals to your brain that promote satiety, slow stomach emptying, and regulate blood sugar.

When you restrict calories, your gut and brain launch a coordinated counterattack. Your gut produces less GLP-1 naturally, weakening the "I'm full" signals sent to your brain. Meanwhile, your brain interprets this as a sign that food is scarce and ramps up reward pathways, making high-calorie foods seem more appealing and harder to resist. This gut-brain communication breakdown is why willpower feels so much harder during dieting. Your brain is literally receiving mixed signals about satisfaction and reward.

How GLP-1 Resets the System

After you eat, your intestine produces GLP-1 to help control blood sugar, signal fullness to your brain, and nudge your body toward healthier metabolism.

Scientists figured out how to create versions of this hormone that work longer and more reliably, giving your system a constant, gentle reminder that you don't need to keep eating nonstop (Strumila et al., 2024).

GLP-1s boost insulin only when your body actually needs it, in direct response to meals. Instead of a flood of insulin every time you eat, your pancreas gets the message to release the right amount. This is a quiet but strong advantage. Less insulin means your body isn't as quick to stash away fat, and your cells process blood sugar more evenly (Strumila et al., 2024).

In daily life, people often notice less of the "energy crash" that can occur a few hours after lunch or a sweet treat. Blood sugar peaks and valleys even out. That steady flow makes it far less likely you'll feel those all-too-familiar swings between cravings, guilt, and fatigue.

Many describe an "appetite reset," in which food thoughts start to settle down. The relentless loop of what to eat, what not to eat, when, and how much loosens its grip. Some notice, often with amazement, that they simply don't finish their meals anymore. A sandwich left half-eaten. A full plate at a birthday party, with no urge to graze mindlessly after. And these aren't fleeting moments of discipline. The effects persist, making portion control effortless instead of exhausting.

Take Margot, a 52-year-old project manager who had struggled with evening binges for years. "Before GLP-1s, I could eat a perfectly balanced dinner and still find myself in the kitchen two hours later, methodically eating through whatever I could find. It wasn't hunger, exactly, but this driving urge that felt impossible to ignore." Within six weeks of starting semaglutide, she noticed a fundamental shift. "I finished half my sandwich at lunch and just... stopped. Not because I was forcing myself to stop, but because I genuinely felt that I was done. For the first time in decades, my body and brain seemed to be having the same conversation about food.

The mental chatter about what to eat next just went quiet." According to clinical findings in European Neuropsychopharmacology, patients treated with GLP-1 receptor agonists consistently report fewer intrusive food thoughts and feel more "in charge" of their hunger (Strumila et al., 2024). Friends and family often notice the change too, meals become about conversation and connection, not a battle against urges or shame.

The benefits extend beyond weight or lab results; GLP-1s help ease decades of self-blame and disappointment that often cling to each new diet or resolution. Years of being told to "just try harder" can leave anyone feeling defeated, as if failure is a result of weak character. Yet biology shapes every step. GLP-1 agonists give proof that your hunger and eating patterns are results of body chemistry, not personality or moral worth.

When a patient says, "For the first time, I could leave food on my plate and not feel deprived," she's rebuilding trust in her body. The cruel voice of self-judgment fades as people realize their struggle was never about laziness or lack of discipline.

The bottom line is that GLP-1 agonists create genuine freedom; the freedom to appreciate yourself as someone shaped by biology, not broken by weakness. The door opens to a new kind of self-esteem, one rooted in kindness toward yourself and a belief in new possibilities for change. Not because you finally found willpower, but because you finally received real support for the way your body truly works.

Breaking Free From Self-Blame

That was the turning point for me: realizing I wasn't just weak, or lazy, or broken beyond repair. My body was running on biology, not willpower. Pain, stress, and years of medications had rewired my system, slowing my metabolism, raising my cortisol, and locking my weight into a higher set point. The science finally gave me the language for what I had been living all along. And once I understood the biology of weight, I could finally stop blaming myself and start focusing on solutions that worked with my body, not against it.

The Stress-Pain-Weight Connection

Chronic pain creates a perfect storm for weight gain and retention. Pain triggers stress responses that elevate cortisol, promote inflammation, and disrupt sleep, all of which make weight loss more difficult. Pain medications can slow metabolism and increase appetite. Limited mobility reduces calorie expenditure and muscle mass.

None of this is a choice or a moral failing. It's physiology responding to circumstances. Understanding this connection allows you to approach weight management with compassion rather than frustration.

Rewriting the Narrative

Instead of "I failed another diet," try "My body's survival mechanisms overpowered my efforts." Instead of "I have no willpower," consider "I was fighting against powerful biological forces without the right tools."

This is not making excuses; it's understanding reality. When you stop wasting energy on self-blame, you can redirect that energy toward strategies that actually work with your biology rather than against it.

Lisa, an accountant who struggled with weight for twenty years, describes her mindset shift: "Once I understood that my hunger and cravings were driven by hormones, not character flaws, everything changed. I stopped seeing myself as broken and started seeing myself as someone who needed the right medical support."

A New Path Forward

Recognizing that biology drives much of our weight regulation doesn't mean giving up, it means getting smarter about our approach. Just as we don't rely on willpower alone to manage diabetes or high blood pressure, we don't have to rely on willpower alone to manage weight.

GLP-1 medications represent a fundamental shift from fighting your body to supporting it. They address the hormonal imbalances that drive hunger and cravings, making sustainable lifestyle changes possible rather than resorting to punishment.

This isn't about taking a pill and ignoring healthy habits. It's about using medical tools to level the playing field, so that eating well and moving more become achievable goals rather than constant struggles against biology.

Understanding your body's weight defense system is the first step toward lasting change. When you stop blaming yourself for biological responses beyond your control, you can start focusing on the tools and strategies that actually work. The next chapter will look more closely into how GLP-1s specifically address these biological challenges, offering hope for a different kind of relationship with food and weight.

Chapter 3:

The Secret Power of GLP-1s: Why They Work When Diets Don't

Three weeks into taking Ozempic, I sat down for lunch and something unexpected happened: I forgot to finish eating. Not because I was distracted or busy, but because my body simply said "enough" halfway through my sandwich. For someone who had spent decades cleaning every plate, this felt revolutionary.

I knew instantly that this wasn't about willpower or discipline. My relationship with hunger itself had fundamentally changed. The medication was working on systems I'd never even known existed, rewiring how my brain and gut communicated about food. Understanding exactly how GLP-1s create this transformation can help you recognize and trust the changes happening in your own body.

This chapter dives into the mechanics behind that transformation. We're going to explore how GLP-1 medications rewire your brain's appetite-control center, stabilize blood sugar to prevent energy crashes, and create lasting changes that feel effortless rather than forced. We'll explore what an "appetite reset" actually feels like day to day, how to adapt your eating patterns to these new signals, and practical strategies for tracking the metabolic improvements that often matter more than the number on the scale.

Your Brain's Appetite Control Center

Deep inside your brain, approximately the size of an almond, sits a region called the hypothalamus that acts as mission control for hunger and appetite. This tiny command center receives constant updates from throughout your body: hormones from your gut reporting what you've eaten, signals from fat cells about energy stores, and messages from your liver about blood sugar levels.

In a healthy system, this information gets processed smoothly. You eat when genuinely hungry, feel satisfied after appropriate portions, and go hours between meals without obsessing about food. But for many of us, especially after years of yo-yo dieting, chronic stress, or metabolic dysfunction, these signals get scrambled.

GLP-1 medications work by strengthening the signal from a specific messenger in this complex system. When you take semaglutide, tirzepatide, or other GLP-1 receptor agonists, you're essentially amplifying the "I'm satisfied" signal that your gut naturally produces after eating. Instead of this message getting lost in the noise, it comes through loud and clear (Mozaffarian et al., 2025).

The "Food Noise" Phenomenon

Many people describe life before GLP-1s as having constant "food noise", a running mental soundtrack of food-related thoughts. What should I eat next? Am I hungry? Should I have a snack? That leftover pizza is calling my name. The bakery smells amazing. Maybe just a small bite.

This mental chatter isn't a character flaw or lack of self-control. Brain imaging studies have shown that individuals with obesity have heightened activity in reward and craving centers when exposed to food cues (Jastreboff et al., 2013; Pursey et al., 2014). Your brain is literally working harder to think about food, making it nearly impossible to focus on anything else for an extended period.

GLP-1 medications quiet this neural static. The constant mental negotiation about food fades into the background. As one patient told me, "I realized I'd gone an entire morning without thinking about lunch. That hadn't happened in years."

Physical Hunger vs. Emotional Eating

It helps to think of hunger as two forces, physical and emotional. GLP-1 medications primarily address one of these but not the other. Physical hunger is your body's biological signal that you need fuel. It builds gradually, can be satisfied with various foods, and resolves after eating.

This is the hunger that GLP-1s help regulate, making it gentler and more manageable.

Emotional eating, on the other hand, often comes on suddenly, craves specific comfort foods (usually sweet, salty, or fatty), and persists even after eating. Sometimes, it actually gets worse. This type of eating is driven by stress, boredom, anxiety, or habit rather than genuine physical need.

So what does this mean practically for you? On GLP-1s, you might find that your 3 p.m. cookie craving (if it was driven by actual hunger) simply disappears. But if you always eat cookies when stressed about work, that urge might persist because it's not really about hunger.

Kiera, a working mother, described this perfectly: "I stopped snacking mindlessly while making dinner for the kids. That was physical hunger, which was satisfied earlier in the day. But I still wanted wine and chocolate after particularly tough bedtime routines. That was stress eating, and the medication didn't touch it."

This distinction is actually helpful. When emotional eating urges arise, you can address them appropriately with stress management techniques, like a phone call to a friend or a short walk, rather than fighting them with willpower.

What an Appetite Reset Actually Feels Like

The "appetite reset" that people talk about isn't a dramatic, overnight change. It's more like someone gradually turning down the volume on a radio that's been too loud for years.

Early Signs of Change

- **Feeling full sooner:** Your usual portion size suddenly feels like too much food.
- **Natural portion control:** You stop eating mid-meal without forcing yourself to stop.
- **Longer periods between meals:** Hours pass without thinking about your next snack.
- **Different relationship with treats:** The office donuts don't call your name as loudly.

Becca a restuarant manager, noticed the shift during family dinners: "I used to serve myself the same portions as my teenage sons and finish everything on my plate.

One evening, I found myself getting up to clear the table while there was still food left on my plate. My husband asked if I was feeling okay, and I realized I just felt satisfied. I wasn't forcing myself to stop eating. I genuinely didn't want any more. After years of either restricting or overeating, this felt like finding a middle ground I'd forgotten existed."

The New Normal

After a few months, many people describe their relationship with food as finally feeling "normal." Meals become fuel and enjoyment rather than constant negotiation. Food remains pleasurable, but it doesn't dominate mental energy.

Don't worry, you won't lose interest in good food or social eating. Instead, you'll be able to enjoy a slice of birthday cake without immediately thinking about having another or splitting an appetizer at dinner because you're genuinely satisfied with less.

Adapting to New Hunger Cues

Learning to trust and respond to your body's new signals takes practice. After years of overriding hunger and fullness cues through restrictive dieting, many people have lost touch with what a normal appetite feels like.

Cue confusion at restaurant tables as a normal portion suddenly feels too much, and the idea of a second helping may seem unthinkable. This reset often brings a gentler, more measured kind of hunger, and satiety signals arrive earlier and more insistently. This is real physiological change, driven by stronger hormonal signaling and less neurochemical reward from eating, so it’s time to trust what your body tells you.

Monitoring Your Fullness

Start paying attention to subtle signs of satisfaction:

- slight pressure in your stomach (not the Thanksgiving-dinner feeling)
- losing interest in the food on your plate
- feeling ready to focus on conversation instead of eating
- a gentle sense of "enough" rather than "stuffed"

Practice the pause: Set your fork down halfway through meals and check in with your body. Are you still hungry, or are you eating from habit?

You can use simple cues throughout your meal. Check in with your body every few bites, and pause halfway through for a thirty-second gut check. If you feel "satisfied" rather than "full," that's your signal to stop, even if there's more food in front of you. Many people notice that they finish half their normal restaurant portion or need to box up leftovers at home, both of which are positive signs that you're listening to your body. This can spark guilt about leaving food behind, but research shows that honoring satiety rather than cleaning your plate helps maintain healthy energy intake and weight (Ciampolini et al., 2013).

Adjusting Meal Timing and Portions

When your hunger starts to dwindle, meal timing becomes really important. It's common to unintentionally skip meals or let hours pass without eating. Set gentle reminders on your phone for regular eating intervals, or schedule meals, such as a protein-rich breakfast, a midday protein snack, and a modest dinner.

Focus on plate balance, not just size. If your protein portions are too small, boost your nutrition by adding extra vegetables or healthy fats like avocado, seeds, or olive oil. Keep easy-to-digest, nutrient-dense snacks handy, like Greek yogurt, nut butter packets, string cheese, or roasted chickpeas.

At restaurants, you could consider ordering an appetizer instead of an entrée, or share mains to match your new appetite. This aligns your intake with your actual hunger rather than forcing yourself to finish standard portions.

Preventing Undereating

One challenge with GLP-1s is that appetite suppression can be so effective that some people accidentally undereat. This is especially common in the first few months as you're adjusting to new signals.

Signs you might not be eating enough:

- persistent fatigue or brain fog
- hair thinning or brittle nails
- mood changes or irritability
- loss of muscle mass
- difficulty concentrating

You're not trying to eat as little as possible; you're trying to eat the right amount for your body's needs while honoring your new hunger cues. Of all these warning signs, loss of muscle mass deserves special attention. Rapid weight loss on GLP-1s can pull a meaningful portion of that loss from lean tissue rather than fat — which is why protein intake and resistance training matter more on these medications than on any diet you've tried. We'll come back to this in Chapter 9 with a practical plan for protecting muscle while the fat comes off.

Blood Sugar Control: The Hidden Benefit

While appetite suppression gets most of the attention, the effects of GLP-1s on blood sugar might be even more significant for long-term health. This is where these medications really shine compared to traditional weight loss approaches.

How GLP-1s Regulate Glucose

Your body's blood sugar regulation system is incredibly sophisticated. After you eat, blood glucose levels rise, triggering the release of insulin to help cells absorb the sugar for energy. GLP-1s enhance this system in several ways (Olukorode et al., 2024; Prasad-Reddy & Isaacs, 2015):

- **Glucose-dependent insulin release:** GLP-1s signal your pancreas to release insulin only when blood sugar levels are elevated. This means no dangerous low blood sugar episodes that can happen with other diabetes medications.
- **Glucagon suppression:** These medications also suppress glucagon, a hormone that tells your liver to dump stored sugar into the bloodstream. By reducing inappropriate glucagon release, GLP-1s prevent unnecessary blood sugar spikes.
- **Slower gastric emptying:** Food moves more slowly from your stomach to your small intestine, leading to more gradual glucose absorption and steadier blood sugar levels throughout the day.

The Dual Benefit: Weight Loss Plus Metabolic Health

What makes GLP-1s uniquely powerful is that they address two interconnected problems simultaneously. Traditional weight loss methods often come at the cost of metabolic health, think crash diets that spike cortisol or extreme restriction that disrupts hormones. However, GLP-1s improve both weight and metabolic function.

For people with prediabetes or type 2 diabetes, this dual action can be life-changing. As weight decreases, insulin sensitivity improves, creating a positive feedback loop. Lower weight means less insulin resistance, which makes further weight loss easier and blood sugar control more stable. Clinical studies consistently show (Olukorode et al., 2024; Prasad-Reddy & Isaacs, 2015):

- **A1C improvements:** Most people see their A1C (average blood sugar over two to three months) drop by one to two percentage points, often moving them from the diabetic to the prediabetic range, or from the prediabetic to the normal range.

- **Fasting glucose reduction:** Morning blood sugar levels typically improve by 20–40 mg/dL, reducing the dawn phenomenon that many diabetics struggle with.
- **Reduced diabetes complications:** Better blood sugar control dramatically lowers the risk of serious complications like neuropathy (nerve damage), retinopathy (eye damage), kidney disease, and cardiovascular problems. Even a 1% reduction in A1C can cut the risk of microvascular complications by up to 37% (Riddle et al., 2018)."

This metabolic improvement often means a reduction in medication. Many people find that their doctors can lower doses of other diabetes medications or eliminate them entirely as their blood sugar stabilizes naturally.

Case in point: one patient started GLP-1 therapy with an A1C of 8.5%. After six months, with fifteen pounds down and little change to the everyday routine, A1C had dropped to 7.1%. Their doctor reduced their blood pressure medications and told them to log their blood sugar half as often. Another example comes from people who have undiagnosed diabetes but live with relentless fatigue and brain fog after meals. After joining a GLP-1 trial, one woman shared she could finally make it through afternoon meetings without zoning out or reaching for caffeine. Her post-lunch crashes vanished, and she was able to keep up with her workout routine much more easily.

Real-World Benefits

Even for those of us without diabetes, GLP-1s can change everyday life. After several weeks, most people notice

- no more afternoon crashes after lunch.
- steadier energy throughout the day.
- less brain fog and better concentration.
- fewer sugar cravings as blood sugar stays stable.
- better sleep without nighttime hunger or energy spikes.

Tracking Your Progress

Keeping track of these changes matters as much as taking the medicine itself. Monitoring your blood sugar improvements can be incredibly motivating.

Below are some ways you can do this:

- **Continuous glucose monitors:** Devices like Dexcom or FreeStyle Libre display real-time glucose readings, allowing you to see how different foods and activities affect your glucose levels.
- **Lab tests:** Your doctor will track A1C (which, as mentioned previously, reflects your average blood sugar over the past two to three months), fasting glucose, and sometimes insulin levels.
- **Apps and tracking:** Use MyFitnessPal, Apple Health, or glucose-specific apps to log readings and spot patterns over time.

While weight loss gets the attention, many people find that steady energy, mental clarity, and freedom from afternoon crashes feel even more transformative than the numbers on the scale. Always keep in mind that these metabolic changes take time to fully develop. Some people notice steadier energy within days, while A1C improvements typically show up after 8–12 weeks. Be patient with the process and celebrate the small wins, such as sleeping better, thinking more clearly, or going hours without thinking about snacks. These are all signs that your body's systems are rebalancing themselves.

Why GLP-1s Succeed Where Diets Fail

Here's what this chapter boils down to: Traditional diets work against your biology, creating an internal battle between willpower and powerful hunger hormones. GLP-1s work with your biology, restoring a more normal appetite and glucose regulation.

This biological approach explains why people can maintain weight loss on GLP-1s without the constant struggle that characterizes traditional dieting. Instead of fighting your body, you're supporting it. The key insight I want you to take with you is that sustainable weight management isn't about having more discipline than the next person, but having the right tools to work with your body's natural systems rather than against them.

Understanding how GLP-1s create these changes helps you trust the process when appetite shifts or blood sugar stabilizes. These are fundamental improvements in how your body regulates energy and hunger. In the next chapter, we will unpack the practical details of different GLP-1 medications, helping you understand which options might work best for your specific situation and goals.

Chapter 4:

Ozempic, Wegovy, Mounjaro, and More

When I first started researching GLP-1 medications, the names felt like alphabet soup. Ozempic, Wegovy, Mounjaro, Trulicity... They all seemed to promise similar results, but the prices and availability varied significantly. Without insurance at the time, cost became my primary concern. That's how I landed on Ozempic, not because it was necessarily the "best" option, but because it was the one I could actually afford and access consistently.

So, I chose Ozempic. Even though it wasn't the highest-dose option, I still started losing weight within a month. For me, accessibility mattered just as much as the science, and that's what made Ozempic the right choice.

This chapter breaks down the major players in the GLP-1 space, helping you understand not only what each medication does, but also how they fit into real-world scenarios such as insurance battles, supply shortages, and personal tolerance. Because the "best" medication is often the one you can actually get and afford to stay on.

Comparing Major GLP-1 Medications

All GLP-1 medications work on the same basic principle: They mimic a hormone your gut naturally produces to regulate appetite and blood sugar. But the details matter when you're choosing which one to take for potentially years. For anyone scanning the shelves at a pharmacy or scrolling through telehealth apps, Ozempic, Wegovy, and Mounjaro look almost identical at first glance. Yet each one is crafted for a different purpose, with unique FDA approvals, active ingredients, dosing plans, and quirks that shape daily life.

Sorting out these medications means answering a few big questions: What's the medicine actually for? What's inside the pen? How often do you need to use it? And perhaps most importantly, what will this mean for routines, results, and out-of-pocket bills?

Let's break them down.

Semaglutide: The Versatile Option

Ozempic and Wegovy both contain semaglutide, but they're approved for different purposes and come in different strengths. Ozempic received FDA approval first, specifically for the management of type 2 diabetes. It's dosed weekly, starting at 0.25 mg and typically maxing out at 2 mg. Many doctors prescribe it "off-label" for weight loss, which is completely legal and common, but insurance coverage can be hit-or-miss for non-diabetic patients (Drugs.com, 2025).

Wegovy contains the same active ingredient but is specifically approved for weight management. The dose increases to 2.4 mg weekly, and the titration schedule is designed to minimize side effects while maximizing weight loss. It's also approved for adolescents aged 12 and up who meet specific criteria (Drugs.com, 2025; Latif et al., 2024).

Drawbacks include the same weekly schedule, some stomach upset, and challenges getting insurance coverage for weight loss; coverage varies widely by plan. For those who want to avoid needles, there's no way around it. Wegovy, like Ozempic, is an injection given in the skin of the belly, thigh, or upper arm once each week. Rybelsus is the oral version of semaglutide, taken daily as a pill. It's convenient for people who hate needles, but the absorption can be tricky—you have to take it on an empty stomach first thing in the morning and wait 30 minutes before eating or drinking anything else (*Rybelsus Dosage Guide*, 2024).

Tirzepatide: The Newcomer With Dual Action

Mounjaro (and its weight-loss branded version Zepbound) contains tirzepatide, which targets both GLP-1 and GIP receptors. This dual action often leads to greater weight loss and improved blood sugar control, but it can also cause more severe side effects. People often report more nausea, vomiting, or digestive discomfort compared with standard semaglutide injectables. For some, this goes away in weeks, but others might need to lower the dose or stop (Drugs.com, 2025).

The dosing schedule is similar to Ozempic, with weekly injections starting at a low dose and titrating up, but the maximum doses are higher, and the effects can be more pronounced. Insurance coverage varies; some plans are slow to cover Mounjaro for weight loss, so readers may face hurdles getting a prescription filled at an affordable rate (Drugs.com, 2025; Latif et al., 2024).

Other Options

Trulicity (dulaglutide) is another weekly injection that some people tolerate better than semaglutide options. Victoza (liraglutide) requires daily injections but has been around longer and has extensive safety data.

Comparing Effectiveness

The numbers from clinical trials tell part of the story, but real-world results can vary significantly based on individual factors.

Weight Loss Results

In clinical studies:

- **Ozempic:** average 12-15% body weight loss over 56 weeks (Kumar & Aronne, 2024; Mozaffarian et al., 2025)
- **Wegovy:** average 15-17% body weight loss over 68 weeks (*Managing Weight with Wegovy*, n.d.)
- **Mounjaro:** average 16-21% body weight loss over 72 weeks (highest doses) (Puddick, 2025)

These are averages, meaning some people lose much more than others. Your results will depend on your starting weight, other health conditions, diet quality, activity level, and how well you tolerate the medication.

Blood Sugar Control

For people with diabetes or prediabetes:

- **Ozempic:** A1C reduction of 1.5-2.0% (Capehorn et al., 2020; Perreault et al., 2022)
- **Mounjaro:** A1C reduction of 2.0-2.4% (Anderson & Marrs, 2023; Eli Lilly, 2025)
- **Wegovy:** similar to Ozempic since it's the same medication (Billingsley, 2022; Stanford, 2025)

These improvements often mean people can reduce or eliminate other diabetes medications, thereby offsetting some of the cost of GLP-1 therapy.

Side Effects and Tolerability

The most common side effects across all GLP-1 medications are gastrointestinal: nausea, vomiting, diarrhea, and constipation. But there are some differences worth noting. Mounjaro tends to cause more intense GI effects (Reynolds, 2025). Because it targets two hormone systems instead of one, tirzepatide often causes stronger side effects, especially during dose escalation.

However, many people find these effects manageable and worth it for the enhanced results. The risk of these symptoms typically increases with higher dosing. People prone to migraines, motion sickness, or GI issues such as IBS may want to start at lower doses or consider dulaglutide or oral medications, which some tolerate better.

Oral semaglutide (Rybelsus) may cause different issues. Some people experience fewer GI side effects with the oral version, while others find the strict dosing requirements (administered on an empty stomach and requiring a 30-minute wait) difficult to maintain consistently (*Semaglutide (Oral Route)*, n.d.).

Fatigue or headache happens less often, and rare risks, like gallbladder disease, pancreatitis, or even hair loss, get more coverage on social media than in clinical care, but they should not be ignored. For anyone with a prior history of gallstones or pancreatitis, it's important to discuss the risk-benefit balance with a healthcare provider (Mozaffarian et al., 2025).

Individual variation is huge. Some people sail through dose increases with minimal side effects, while others need to go very slowly or switch medications entirely. This isn't predictable based on age, weight, or other factors; it's simply a matter of individual body chemistry.

The Cost Reality

Here's where the rubber meets the road for most people. Out-of-pocket pricing for branded drugs is steep: Ozempic and Wegovy often run $900 to $1,300 per month if insurance doesn't help, and Mounjaro ranges from $1,000 to $1,300. With commercial insurance, monthly copays can range from $25 to $75, but this depends on both plan generosity and "step therapy" policies that may require trialing cheaper drugs first.

Medicare and Medicaid access can be hit-or-miss, since weight loss is not always a covered indication. Manufacturer savings programs or coupons help, but they rarely cover those on government health plans.

Insurance Coverage Strategies

For diabetes: Ozempic and Mounjaro are typically well-covered since they're approved for diabetes management.

For weight loss: Coverage is inconsistent. Wegovy and Zepbound are specifically approved for weight management, but many insurance plans don't cover weight loss medications at all.

Off-label prescribing: Your doctor can prescribe Ozempic for weight loss, even if you don't have diabetes; however, insurance coverage becomes less predictable.

Compounded Alternatives

When brand-name medications are unavailable or unaffordable, some people turn to compounded versions from specialty pharmacies. These typically cost $200-400 per month but come with important caveats:

- Quality varies between compounding pharmacies.
- There is no FDA oversight of the final product.
- There are legal gray areas around certain formulations.

- Supply can be unreliable.

If you're considering compounded medications, work with a reputable pharmacy and a knowledgeable healthcare provider.

Considering these choices matters because the numbers only tell part of the story. Behind every script and insurance card is a person juggling work schedules, family demands, and their own vision for long-term health.

Real-World Switching Stories

The decision to switch medications is rarely based solely on effectiveness, it's usually driven by access, cost, or tolerability issues.

From Ozempic to Mounjaro

Eve, a 45-year-old teacher, started on Ozempic through her doctor's samples. "I lost 25 pounds in four months and felt great, but when the samples ran out, my insurance wouldn't cover it for weight loss. My doctor suggested Mounjaro since it was covered for my prediabetes.

The transition was rough, with much more nausea and fatigue for the first month. However, once I adjusted, I actually came to prefer it. The appetite suppression was stronger, and my blood sugar numbers improved more than they had on Ozempic."

From Wegovy to Compounded Semaglutide

Hamil, a small business owner, faced a different challenge: "Wegovy was working amazingly. I lost 40 pounds in six months. But the pharmacy kept having shortages, and I'd go weeks without medication. Every time I stopped and restarted, the side effects came back full force. I switched to compounded semaglutide from a local pharmacy. It's not exactly the same, but it's consistent, and I can afford it without insurance coverage."

Finding the Right Fit

Lauren tried three different options before finding her match: "Ozempic made me constantly nauseous. Wegovy was better but expensive. Mounjaro gave me terrible fatigue. Finally tried Trulicity, and while the weight loss was slower, I felt like myself again.

Sometimes the best medication is the one you can actually live with."

Making Your Choice

The "best" GLP-1 medication depends on several factors:

Your Primary Goal

- **Blood sugar control:** Ozempic or Mounjaro is typically covered by insurance.
- **Weight loss:** Wegovy or Zepbound is designed specifically for this purpose.
- **Both:** Mounjaro/Zepbound often provide the strongest effects for both goals.

Your Insurance Situation

- **Good coverage:** Go with what's covered and see how you respond.
- **Limited coverage:** Consider off-label prescribing of Ozempic or Mounjaro.
- **No coverage:** Explore manufacturer programs, compounded options, or clinical trials.

Your Tolerance for Side Effects

- **Sensitive stomach:** Start with Ozempic or consider Trulicity.
- **Want maximum results:** Try Mounjaro despite potentially stronger side effects.

- **Hate needles:** If you hate needles, try Rybelsus, understanding the dosing requirements.

Your Lifestyle

- **Travel frequently:** Weekly injections are more convenient than daily pills.
- **Irregular schedule:** Daily pills might be easier to remember.
- **Want simplicity:** Stick with whatever you can access consistently.

Working With Your Healthcare Provider

The decision shouldn't be made in isolation. A good healthcare provider will consider

- your medical history and current medications.
- your weight loss and health goals.
- your insurance coverage and financial situation.
- your previous experiences with medications.
- monitoring requirements and follow-up plans.

Don't hesitate to advocate for yourself if cost or access is an issue. Most providers understand these practical constraints and can work with you to find solutions.

The goal is finding a medication that works for your body, your budget, and your life. Sometimes that means starting with what's available and adjusting later. Other times, it means holding out for the option that best fits your specific situation.

Making It Work for You

Choosing the right GLP-1 medication isn't a one-size-fits-all decision. What works for your neighbor might not work for you, and what's covered by your insurance might not be the most effective option for your body. The key is finding the balance between clinical effectiveness, practical accessibility, and your own tolerance and lifestyle needs.

Don't be discouraged if your first choice isn't perfect. Many people try multiple medications before finding their ideal match, and switching between GLP-1s is common and safe when done under medical supervision. Your needs may also change over time; what works during the initial weight loss phase might need adjustment for long-term maintenance.

Remember, these medications work best as part of a comprehensive approach that includes attention to nutrition, movement, sleep, and stress management. The medication creates the biological conditions for success, but lasting change requires building sustainable habits around those improvements.

The most important factor is consistency. The best GLP-1 medication is the one you can access reliably, afford sustainably, and tolerate well enough to stay on long-term. Perfect shouldn't be the enemy of good when it comes to your health.

In the next chapter, we'll dive into the practical aspects of getting started with whichever medication you and your provider decide is right for you, from navigating insurance approvals to preparing for your first injection.

Chapter 5:

Starting Your GLP-1 Journey With Confidence

Walking into a doctor's office to discuss GLP-1 medications can feel intimidating, especially if you've had dismissive experiences in the past. Maybe you've sat through appointments where your weight concerns were brushed off with generic advice about eating less and moving more. Or perhaps you've felt judged for wanting medical help rather than relying solely on willpower.

I remember my first conversation with my doctor about Ozempic. I'd done my homework, gathered my medical history, and prepared my questions, but I still felt nervous. Would he take me seriously? Would insurance cover it? What if he said no?

Preparation made all the difference. By the time I left that appointment, I had a prescription, a clear plan for managing side effects, and the documentation needed for insurance approval. This chapter will provide you with the tools to have that same kind of productive conversation, navigate the insurance maze, and start your GLP-1 journey with confidence.

Why Self-Advocacy Matters

Nobody walks into their provider's office hoping to feel lost, rushed, or dismissed. It's normal to experience uncertainty or even anxiety before a major health conversation, especially when you're navigating midlife shifts, new symptoms, or a history of "not quite fitting" typical treatment boxes.

Will the doctor think I'm vain or impatient? Will I leave with the same old advice?

Whether they're related to long-term weight struggles, changes during menopause, skeptical providers, or complicated insurance paperwork, when your concerns run deep, it's easy to feel like you're advocating for more than just a prescription. You're actually standing up for your well-being in a medical system that sometimes moves too fast to see the full you.

Self-advocacy doesn't mean you need to be confrontational or demanding. It means coming prepared, asking informed questions, and ensuring your healthcare provider has the complete picture of your health journey. When you advocate effectively for yourself, you create a partnership with your provider rather than a one-sided consultation.

Healthcare providers see dozens of patients each week, often with limited time per appointment. The more organized and informed you are, the more likely you are to get the attention and care you deserve. This is especially important for GLP-1 medications, which many providers are still learning about and which require specific documentation for insurance approval.

Patients who come prepared with organized medical histories and clear questions tend to have better outcomes and higher satisfaction with their care. They're also more likely to be approved for newer treatments like GLP-1 therapy because they can demonstrate medical necessity effectively.

Preparing for Your Appointment

Preparatory work makes a difference in both your results and your emotional experience.

Organizing Your Medical History

Before your visit, gather recent lab results; notes from any prior discussions about weight, blood sugar, or metabolic health; and a list of every medication, supplement, and over-the-counter therapy you take. If you've tracked your food, exercise, or blood sugars at home, bring that documentation, too. Gather all relevant medical records from the past three years.

- **Lab results:** recent A1C, fasting glucose, lipid panels, kidney function tests, and thyroid function

- **Medication history:** current prescriptions, supplements, and any medications you've tried and stopped
- **Previous weight loss attempts:** documented programs, medications, or supervised diet plans
- **Health conditions:** diabetes, prediabetes, high blood pressure, sleep apnea, PCOS, or other metabolic conditions
- **Family history:** diabetes, heart disease, obesity, or other relevant conditions

Documentation That Strengthens Your Case

Jot down your previous approaches to weight or glucose management, including any diet plans, physical activity routines, behavioral changes, support groups, even if they didn't lead to lasting changes. The more complete a picture you can provide, the more your provider can work with you. Create a simple timeline of your weight and health journey. For example:

- **2020:** Started Weight Watchers, lost 15 pounds over 6 months, regained 18 pounds by the end of the year.
- **2021:** Tried intermittent fasting for 4 months, lost 8 pounds, but couldn't maintain due to work schedule.
- **2022:** Started metformin for prediabetes, A1C improved from 6.2% to 5.9%.
- **2023:** Attempted keto diet, lost 12 pounds in 3 months, experienced fatigue, and stopped.

Insurance companies often require proof of "failed conservative management" before approving GLP-1 medications. Document each of your previous attempts with the following:

- program name and duration
- amount of weight lost and regained
- reasons for discontinuation
- any side effects or challenges

Keep records of any medically supervised attempts, as these carry more weight with insurance companies than self-directed efforts.

Organizing Your Documentation Effectively

Having your information organized not only shows professionalism but also strengthens self-advocacy.

When a provider sees that you've prepared purposefully, the dynamic shifts, and you are no longer a passive recipient but an active collaborator in your care.

Creating a Detailed Medications List

Start by assembling a complete medication list that includes the name of each medication, the prescribed dose, whether it is a brand or generic, when you started taking it, and any side effects or allergic reactions.

Here's a simple format:

Medication name	Dose	Brand/generic	Start date	Reason	Noted side effects
e.g. Metformin	1000 mg	Generic	Jan 2022	T2D	Mild upset stomach

A printout like this, or a screenshot from your phone's health app, reduces confusion and helps your provider understand your complete treatment history.

Documenting Your Weight Loss History

Insurance companies often require proof of "medically-supervised" attempts before approving GLP-1 therapy.

Document each attempt using this format:

Diet program	Start/end	Adherence	Outcome	Notes
Mediterranean Diet	February 2021–May 2021	Tracked meals 5-6 days/week; followed plan at least 80% of the time	Lost 7 pounds; regained 6 pounds by July 2021	Struggled with evening cravings, stress eating after work

Include programs such as Weight Watchers, intermittent fasting, keto, or any prescription medications you have tried. If a medication caused side effects, note them clearly. Also document personal challenges that affect weight management, such as menopause, thyroid changes, mobility issues, or major life transitions.

Gathering Health Records

Collect recent lab results, including A1C, fasting glucose, lipid panels, kidney function, and thyroid tests. If you use health apps or continuous glucose monitors, prepare summaries showing patterns over the last 6-12 months. Platforms like MyChart or Apple Health make it easy to export official results.

Creating Your Appointment Checklist

Prepare a checklist with headings like:

- Key Questions for My Doctor
- Insurance Info to Bring
- Recent Lab Results & Dates
- GLP-1 Goals and Concerns

Journaling Your Health Story

Spend five minutes answering these prompts:

- "How have weight and metabolic health impacted my quality of life?"
- "What has been my biggest challenge with past diets?"
- "How do I want GLP-1 therapy to improve my daily functioning?"

These personal notes help translate clinical numbers into a real-life context and show your provider why you're committed to this process.

During the Appointment

This is the big moment. Take a deep breath before you do anything else and believe in all the prep work you've been doing.

Starting the Conversation

When you're ready, introduce your records at the beginning of your appointment. Try beginning by saying something like, "I've put together my history so you can get the full picture of where I'm coming from and what I've already tried," or "I know I'm asking about something new; here's my background so we can make the best choice together." This approach demonstrates thoughtfulness and builds trust, showing you're invested in your health.

The conversation about GLP-1 medications works even better with a prepared opener. Some like a direct approach, such as, "Based on my history and what I've read, I want to discuss whether a GLP-1 could be a fit for me."

Those who prefer collaboration might try, "I'm interested in talking through options like GLP-1s. Would you help me understand where they could fit into my care?" If you're inquisitive, you might ask, "What are your thoughts on GLP-1 medications for someone with my health background?" These scripts allow space for dialogue and signal openness to professional advice.

Essential Questions to Ask

Talking through the available choices means exploring the details, so it can help to bring up specific questions about GLP-1 therapy. Ask about the different GLP-1 options and how they compare in effectiveness, lifestyle impact, and side effects.

Questions for your provider might include:

About the medication:

- Which GLP-1 medication do you recommend for my situation and why?
- How does this interact with my current medications?
- What side effects should I expect, and how can I manage them?
- How will we monitor my progress?

About logistics:

- What's the typical timeline for insurance approval?
- Are there manufacturer savings programs I should know about?
- How often will I need follow-up appointments?
- What should I do if I experience concerning side effects?

About alternatives:

- What other options exist if this doesn't work for me?
- Are there lifestyle modifications that would enhance the medication's effectiveness?
- What's your experience prescribing these medications?

Your next steps depend on the groundwork you lay now. Gather your medical records, outline your medication trials, and think through the questions and scripts that fit your voice.

With this toolkit, you're setting yourself up for a visit that's informed, respectful, and centered on partnership, setting a foundation for the rest of your GLP-1 journey.

When Your Provider Is Hesitant

Not all healthcare providers are comfortable prescribing GLP-1 medications for weight loss. Some may be unfamiliar with the latest research, concerned about side effects, or have personal biases about weight management medications.

Addressing Common Concerns

"You should try diet and exercise first."

Response: "I've documented several supervised attempts at diet and lifestyle modification. Here's my history of what I've tried and the outcomes. I'm looking for tools to help make sustainable lifestyle changes more achievable."

"These medications are too new/risky."

Response: "Can you help me understand your specific concerns? I've seen that semaglutide has been used for diabetes management since 2017 and has extensive safety data. What additional information would help you feel more comfortable?"

"Insurance won't cover it anyway."

Response: "I understand coverage can be challenging. Would you be willing to prescribe it with proper documentation so we can at least try the insurance approval process? I'm prepared to explore other payment options if needed."

When to Seek a Second Opinion

If your provider remains reluctant despite your preparation and documented medical necessity, it may be time to seek care elsewhere. Consider:

- endocrinologists who specialize in diabetes and metabolism
- weight management clinics or bariatric medicine specialists
- internal medicine physicians with experience in obesity medicine
- telemedicine platforms that specialize in GLP-1 prescribing

Don't take a "no" personally. Some providers simply aren't comfortable with newer treatments, and that's okay. Your goal is to find someone who can partner with you effectively.

Navigating Insurance Approvals

Just as with your provider, holding organized records—such as medication lists, a calendar of past weight management methods, and notes about your journey—gives you vital leverage during the insurance approval process.

Understanding Prior Authorization

Most insurance plans require prior authorization for GLP-1 medications, especially when they are prescribed for weight loss.

The step from personal organization to successful authorization for GLP-1 prescriptions starts with presenting a detailed, real story that supports your medical necessity and readiness to commit. Insurance plans require more than just a prescription. They require proof that this medication meets their "clinical criteria," demonstrating the necessity and the absence of better alternatives for you (Bertagna, 2024).

This process typically involves

1. the initial prescription submission by your provider.
2. an insurance review of medical necessity criteria.
3. a request for additional documentation if needed.
4. an approval or denial decision (usually within 15-30 days).
5. an appeals process if initially denied.

Key Documentation for Approval

When your provider submits a prior authorization for a GLP-1, your insurance company checks if your case meets their "clinical criteria." These rules outline who qualifies for coverage, often requiring BMI minimums, a record of failed weight-loss attempts, and proof that the medication will treat or prevent other health problems.

"Documentation" is the medical paperwork that supports your doctor's request: clinic visits, failed weight loss methods, reports of side effects from earlier drugs, and lab tests.

"Medical necessity" is a term insurers use for treatments considered crucial for your health, something both you and your physician will need to prove.

Checklist: What to Gather and Submit

- provider's prescription for a GLP-1
- documentation of failed first-line treatments like diet, exercise, or other weight loss drugs
- laboratory results that reveal related health risks or show previous medication effects
- evidence of existing medical conditions that are affected by weight (like high blood pressure or diabetes)
- doctor's statement describing the need for treatment: why alternatives failed, what you hope to accomplish, and the harms of leaving obesity untreated
- your personal account: a short summary of your experience and goals, especially how your weight impacts daily life

Expect the insurance company to ask for this information within a few days to a few weeks. They may take 15–30 business days to review your case, but delays are common (Bertagna, 2024).

Sample Scripts and Letters

Preparing scripts can help your conversations go smoothly and focus everyone's attention. When speaking to your provider, try, "I'd like to pursue GLP-1 therapy, and I have documented attempts and outcomes from previous treatments. Can you help me submit prior authorization with these details?" If your insurer calls or emails, say, "I want to confirm you received the full set of documentation for my prior authorization. Could you clarify if more information is needed?"

A sample doctor's letter of medical necessity may read:

"To whom it may concern,

My patient [Name] is a [age]-year-old with a BMI of [number] and a history of [relevant conditions]. Despite multiple documented attempts at lifestyle modification, including [list programs/medications], the patient has been unable to achieve sustained weight loss. Current weight significantly affects [specific health conditions/quality-of-life issues]. Based on clinical guidelines and evidence supporting GLP-1 therapy for obesity management, I recommend [specific medication] as medically necessary for this patient's health and well-being."

If your initial request is denied, you can write your own appeal:

"Dear [Insurance Company],

I am writing to appeal the denial of coverage for [GLP-1 medication] under claim number [number].

My medical history includes [relevant conditions], and I have made multiple documented attempts at weight management, including [list attempts with dates and outcomes]. These conservative measures have not resulted in sustained weight loss, and my current weight continues to negatively impact my health through [specific examples].

[Medication name] is FDA-approved for my condition and is considered appropriate treatment per current medical guidelines. My physician has determined this medication is medically necessary based on my individual health profile and treatment history.

I respectfully request reconsideration of this denial and approval of coverage for this medically necessary treatment.

Sincerely, [Your name]"

Key phrases that help include:

- evidence-based
- failed first-line options
- documented side effects
- FDA-approved for this indication
- impact on daily function
- risk reduction for future complications

These terms match what insurers look for to justify an exception or approve a treatment request (Pollock, 2024; Bertagna, 2024).

Advocating for Medication Switches

If you're already on a GLP-1 but experiencing problematic side effects or cost issues, you may need to advocate for switching to a different option. This requires a different approach than initial prescribing.

- **For side effect issues:** "I've been on [current medication] for [timeframe] and while I'm seeing [positive results], I'm experiencing [specific side effects] that are impacting my daily life. Can we discuss switching to [alternative medication] that might be better tolerated?"
- **For cost issues:** "My insurance situation has changed, and [current medication] is no longer affordable. Based on my response to this medication, what similar options might have better coverage or lower costs?"
- **For effectiveness concerns:** "I've been on [current medication] for [timeframe] at the maximum dose, but my progress has stalled. Are there other GLP-1 options that might be more effective for my situation?"

Key strategies:

- Document the specific problems you're experiencing (side effect frequency, financial impact, lack of progress).
- Research which alternatives might address your concerns.
- Ask about the timing of switching and whether you need to taper off the current medication.
- Request documentation from your insurance provider that explains the medical necessity of the switch.

Your provider should be willing to work with you on switching medications, especially if you can demonstrate that the current medication isn't meeting your needs despite adequate trial duration.

When Coverage Is Denied

Don't give up after an initial denial.

Options include:

Immediate steps:

- Request a detailed explanation of the denial reason.
- Work with your provider to address any missing documentation.
- File a formal appeal within the specified timeframe.

Financial assistance:

- Manufacturer savings programs (often $25-150/month with commercial insurance).
- Pharmacy discount cards (e.g., GoodRx, SingleCare).
- Patient assistance programs for those who qualify financially.

Alternative approaches:

- Ask about different GLP-1 medications that might have better coverage.
- Consider compounded semaglutide from specialty pharmacies.
- Explore clinical trials in your area.

Staying Persistent and Empowered

The Appeals Process

If your initial request is denied, don't take it as a final answer. The appeals process exists because insurance companies often deny claims that should be approved. Key strategies:

- **Document everything:** Keep detailed records of all communications, reference numbers, and timelines.
- **Follow up regularly:** Don't assume silence means progress.
- **Escalate when necessary:** Request peer-to-peer reviews where a physician reviews your case.
- **Know your timeline:** Most appeals have specific deadlines that must be met.

Working with Your Healthcare Team

Your provider's office can be your biggest ally in the insurance process. Many organizations have staff dedicated to prior authorizations who are well-versed in the system. Don't hesitate to do the following:

- Ask about their experience with GLP-1 approvals.
- Request updates on your case status.
- Ask them to call the insurance company directly if there are delays.

Managing Expectations and Staying Motivated

The approval process can be frustrating and time-consuming. Frame setbacks as "not no, just not yet" rather than permanent roadblocks. Many people who are initially denied eventually get approved through persistence and proper documentation.

Remember that this process is an investment in your long-term health. The effort you put in now to navigate insurance and find the right provider will pay off when you're successfully managing your weight and improving your metabolic health.

When to Escalate Further

If standard appeals aren't working:

- Contact your state's insurance commissioner if you believe your denial was inappropriate.
- Work with your HR department if you have employer-sponsored insurance.
- Consider consulting a lawyer for cases involving clear insurance bad faith.
- Document patterns if you notice your insurance company systematically denying appropriate claims.

Getting Started Once Approved

Once you have approval and your prescription, you're ready to begin. Your provider should give you

- clear instructions for the injection technique and timing.
- information about expected side effects and when to call.
- a plan for dose escalation and monitoring.
- resources for ongoing support.

The preparation work you've done will continue to serve you throughout your GLP-1 journey. The organizational skills and self-advocacy strategies that helped you get started will be valuable for ongoing monitoring, dose adjustments, and any challenges that arise.

Moving Forward With Confidence

Starting GLP-1 therapy is a significant step that requires preparation, persistence, and patience. By coming to your appointments organized and informed, advocating clearly for your needs, and understanding the insurance landscape, you set yourself up for success.

This process is about more than just getting a prescription. You're building a foundation for long-term health management and establishing yourself as an active partner in your healthcare. The skills you develop during this process will serve you well throughout your health journey.

In the next chapter, we'll start looking at what to expect during your first 90 days on GLP-1 therapy, including how to manage side effects, track your progress, and build sustainable habits around your new medication routine.

Chapter 6:

The First 90 Days: What to Expect (and What's Totally Normal)

When I took my very first injection, I honestly didn't know what to expect. I was nervous, second-guessing myself, and convinced something was going to go wrong.

In fact, I was so uneasy about the idea of sticking a needle in myself that I asked my partner to do it for me for the first couple of weeks. What surprised me most? There was absolutely no pain. The needle tip is tiny, far smaller than I had imagined—and after a while, it became routine.

Today, some GLP-1 medications even come in pill form instead of injections, which can be a relief for people who can't stand the idea of needles. But for me, once I got past the fear, the weekly injection became surprisingly easy to manage.

By the end of that first week, I noticed something I hadn't experienced before: my appetite had shifted. It was subtle, almost like background "food noise" had quieted down. I wasn't obsessing over my next meal in the same way, and for the first time in years, that gave me a strange but undeniable feeling of hope.

The first 90 days of GLP-1 therapy are less about flawless execution and more about steady discovery. You're learning to listen to your body's new signals, adapting to changes, and building routines that will support your long-term success.

This chapter will guide you through what to expect, how to manage common challenges, and most importantly, how to recognize progress beyond just the number on the scale.

Your First Injection: Day-by-Day Reality

Starting a new GLP-1 medication, whether it's injected or taken by mouth, brings a mix of anticipation and uncertainty. The first month feels like a test run, a time to find your rhythm, notice what your body tells you, and practice giving yourself plenty of grace along the way. You might feel energized to finally take action, but those energetic first days can hit plenty of speed bumps.

People describe feeling curious, hopeful, nervous, or even skeptical, sometimes all in the same morning. Some recount peering anxiously at an injection pen, heart pounding, while others second-guess whether they measured the dose correctly or set their reminder right.

These reactions are completely ordinary, regardless of your background or how detail-oriented you are. Even patients with years of health experience have felt uneasy giving themselves a first shot, worried about doing it wrong, or frustrated by unfamiliar side effects (*Frequently Asked Questions*, 2025). Here, I'll walk you through the day-to-day reality to help you feel prepared and know what to expect.

The Night Before

Many people spend the evening before their first injection reading and re-reading instructions, watching YouTube videos, or texting friends who've been through this. That nervous energy is completely normal.

You can set yourself up for success by having everything ready: your medication, alcohol wipes, and a calm environment where you won't be rushed or interrupted.

Day One: The First Shot

If you're using an injection pen, here's what actually happens:

1. **Preparation:** Wash your hands, and remove the medication from the refrigerator 15-30 minutes in advance to allow it to reach room temperature. Cold medication can sting more.
2. **Location:** Most people inject into their thighs, upper arms, or stomach areas. Rotate sites to prevent irritation.

3. **The injection:** Remove the pen cap, attach the needle (if separate), dial your dose, insert the needle at a 90-degree angle, press the button firmly, and hold for 10 seconds after the injection completes.
4. **Reality check:** The needle is about as thin as an acupuncture needle. Most people describe it as a small pinch or barely noticeable. The anticipation is almost always worse than the actual injection.

Days 1-3: Initial Responses

Here's what you can expect to feel in those first few days (*Frequently Asked Questions*, 2025; *Improving the Patient Onboarding Experience*, 2024):

- **Appetite changes:** You might notice subtle shifts in hunger. Some people feel less interested in food immediately, while others don't notice changes for several days.
- **Mild nausea:** This is the most common early side effect, often described as similar to mild motion sickness. It typically peaks two to four hours after injection and may last one to two days.
- **Fatigue:** Some people feel slightly tired or "off" for the first few days. This usually resolves as your body adjusts.
- **Injection site:** Minor redness, bruising, or tenderness at the injection site is normal and typically resolves within 24-48 hours.

Days 4-7: Finding Your Rhythm

By the end of the first week, most people start to notice more consistent changes:

- feeling full sooner during meals
- less thinking about food between meals
- possible mild digestive changes
- beginning to establish an injection routine and timing

Common concerns: "Is this working?" "Should I feel more dramatic changes?" "What if I'm not responding?" These doubts are universal. Remember, GLP-1 medications work gradually, not dramatically.

Creating Your Baseline: Tracking What Matters

Moving through the first few weeks of GLP-1 therapy, you might have noticed that emotions can shift day to day, and initial side effects often bring a mix of hopefulness and worry. These early hurdles are not just a challenge to endure. They invite you to notice changes that matter, even if the scale seems stuck or numbers move slowly. Redefining what counts as achievement expands the picture of your progress, making room for victories that fit your life and priorities.

Before you can recognize progress, you need to know where you're starting from. Creating a comprehensive baseline goes far beyond just stepping on a scale. Let's take a look at the kinds of things you can measure and keep track of from day one.

Physical Measures

- **Weight and body metrics:**
    - current weight (same scale, same time of day)
    - waist circumference at the navel level
    - blood pressure if you have a home monitor
    - any measurements you want to track (arms, thighs, etc.)
- **Lab values if available:**
    - A1C and fasting glucose
    - lipid panel (cholesterol, triglycerides)
    - kidney and liver function tests
- **Fitness markers:**
    - daily step count average (use phone or fitness tracker)
    - how many flights of stairs you can climb without stopping
    - how long you can walk at a comfortable pace

Subjective Measures

Success that truly supports your health comes from more than a single measure. Relying solely on body weight can leave you feeling defeated when your hard work is actually paying off in other ways. These "soft" metrics often change before the scale moves and can be incredibly motivating:

- **Energy levels:** Rate your daily energy on a scale of 1-10. Track when you feel most energetic and when you crash.
- **Sleep quality:** Note how long it takes to fall asleep, whether you wake up during the night, and how rested you feel in the morning.
- **Mood and mental clarity:** Track overall mood, anxiety levels, and afternoon brain fog.
- **Hunger and cravings:** Note when you typically get hungry, what you crave, and how strong those cravings feel.
- **Physical comfort:** Joint pain, heartburn, bloating, or other discomforts that might improve with weight loss.

Digital Tools for Tracking

Self-tracking doesn't have to be complicated or time-consuming. Choose one or two practical methods that fit your lifestyle:

- **Smartphone apps:**
    - MyFitnessPal for food logging and basic health metrics
    - Apple Health or Google Fit for automatic activity tracking
    - Mood tracking apps like Daylio or eMoods
    - Sleep tracking through your phone or wearable device
- **Wearable devices:**
    - fitness trackers for steps, heart rate, and sleep
    - continuous glucose monitors if you have diabetes or prediabetes
    - smart scales that track weight trends over time

- **Simple alternatives:**
  - a notebook or journal for daily observations
  - weekly photos in the same outfit and lighting
  - a basic calendar to mark good days vs. challenging days

Seeing your own data plotted over a month or two makes small changes visible and builds confidence. What you gain from fresh routines, meals out with friends, or better sleep lines up as proof of real, day-to-day achievement.

Paying attention to these meaningful markers puts you in a strong position to shape your personal baseline and create routines that work for you, not against you. These ongoing snapshots of progress make it easier to see what's changing and help you stay motivated for everything ahead (Davies et al., 2021; Varajão et al., 2022).

Using Your Baseline for Goal Setting

Once you have your baseline measurements, you can use them to create SMART goals (Specific, Measurable, Achievable, Realistic, Time-bound) that fit your starting point:

Weight-based example: "I will lose 8-12 pounds over the next 12 weeks (1-2 lbs per week average)."

Energy-based example: "I will increase my daily step count from my baseline of 4,000 steps to 6,000 steps by week 8."

Sleep-based example: "I will improve my sleep quality rating from my baseline of 5/10 to 7/10 within six weeks by maintaining consistent bedtimes."

Mood-based example: "I will reduce my afternoon energy crashes from daily (baseline) to two to three times per week within four weeks."

Share these goals and your baseline data with your provider. This collaborative approach helps them understand your priorities and adjust your treatment plan accordingly.

Titration 101: Safely Increasing Your Dose

Most GLP-1 medications start at a low dose and are gradually increased over several weeks or months. This process, known as titration, helps minimize side effects while finding your optimal dose.

Self-tracking gives you a running start not just because when you record symptoms and patterns from day one, you spot both progress and trouble quickly. This habit also becomes the anchor point for every new dose adjustment, making each increase less daunting and more informed.

Why Start Low and Go Slow

GLP-1 medications work best when you increase doses slowly, letting your body get used to each level, because higher doses too soon can crank up nausea or other unwanted effects (Nieuwlaat et al., 2014).

Your digestive system needs time to adjust to the medication's effects. Starting at a high dose dramatically increases the risk of severe nausea, vomiting, and other side effects that might force you to stop the medication entirely.

Typical Titration Schedules

Most titration routines follow either a weekly or biweekly plan. With weekly titration, you might spend seven days at one dose, then bump up to the next level on your regular "shot day." A biweekly plan stretches each step to 14 days, sometimes taking pressure off by giving you more time to settle before making a change. Typical titration calendars look like this: say you start at Dose A on Monday of week one.

If your doctor gives the go-ahead, the following Monday becomes "titration week," where you administer Dose B and continue to log your reactions, energy, and hunger cues as before. If you're moving in two-week intervals, that first Monday is Dose A, and you wait for the second Monday to try Dose B. Not everyone will be ready for each new step on time.

If you notice extra fatigue, ongoing nausea, or anything else causing real discomfort, you're allowed (and encouraged) to stay at the current dose longer. Just note your reasons and check in with your healthcare provider instead of pushing onward too soon.

Managing Dose Increases

Every dose change comes with some simple safety steps. First, read the label and the device instructions, double-checking the dose before each shot or pill. If a dose is skipped by mistake, don't double up.

For once-weekly injections, take the missed dose as soon as you remember, provided it's within three days of your usual schedule. If you're already too close to the next scheduled dose, skip the missed dose and continue your regular schedule.

It can be helpful to use a digital tracking app, a recurring calendar alert, or even a paper "dose log" taped to the fridge to help prevent missed doses. Many people find that setting a recurring morning phone alert with a special sound or color-coding a pill organizer helps lock in the routine.

Before making a dose change, keep records of your appetite, GI symptoms, and energy levels, as these are what your provider will want to know. Safe medication relies on honesty about what you've noticed. Any time you experience severe vomiting, fainting, signs of dehydration, or trouble breathing, reach out to your care team immediately, as these are all signals that you need help that can't wait.

Write down any questions you might have, such as: "What should I do if the nausea gets worse?" or "How do I know if it's time to pause dose increases?" and bring your symptom logs to every follow-up visit (Nieuwlaat et al., 2014).

- **Before each increase:**
    - Review your symptom log with your provider.
    - Ensure current side effects are manageable.
    - Discuss any concerns or questions.
- **After each increase**:
    - Monitor for new or worsening side effects.

    - Track appetite and digestive changes.
    - Don't hesitate to slow down if needed.
- **When to pause or reduce:**
    - Persistent vomiting that prevents eating or drinking.
    - Severe fatigue that interferes with daily activities.
    - Any side effect that feels unmanageable.

There's no prize for reaching the highest dose quickly. The goal is to find the dose that gives you good results with tolerable side effects.

Finding Your Voice and Community Support

Learning to communicate effectively with your healthcare team becomes crucial during the titration process. Don't minimize your symptoms or tough it out unnecessarily.

Be specific when reporting side effects: "I'm experiencing nausea three to four hours after injection that lasts about 18 hours and makes it difficult to eat more than a few bites" is more helpful than "I feel sick."

Many people find peer support invaluable during this adjustment period. Online communities, such as Reddit's r/Semaglutide or Facebook groups dedicated to GLP-1 medications, offer real-world insights and encouragement.

Jessica, a marketing coordinator, found community support essential: "Week 3 was brutal—constant nausea, and I was convinced I'd have to quit. Reading stories from people who pushed through similar experiences and felt better by week 5 gave me the courage to call my doctor and slow down the titration instead of giving up entirely."

Common peer wisdom you can expect includes: "It gets better after week two," "Don't rush the dose increases," and "Side effects are temporary, benefits last." While every person's experience is different, knowing you're not alone in the struggle helps maintain perspective during difficult adjustment periods.

Your Side Effect Survival Kit

Most people experience some side effects during the first 90 days. Being prepared helps you manage them effectively rather than feeling overwhelmed. Below is an easy-to-use reference guide to help you determine what's normal, what you can expect, and when you need to seek medical help (Nieuwlaat et al., 2014; Aghajanian et al., 2018).

Nausea: The Most Common Challenge

When it typically occurs: two to six hours after injection, lasting one to three days, often worse with dose increases

Management strategies:

- Eat smaller, more frequent meals.
- Avoid greasy, spicy, or high-fat foods.
- Try bland foods: crackers, toast, rice, bananas.
- Ginger tea, ginger chews, or ginger supplements.
- Stay hydrated with small, frequent sips.
- Avoid lying down immediately after eating.

Red flags: persistent vomiting that prevents keeping down fluids for 24+ hours

Constipation: The Overlooked Problem

Why it happens: GLP-1s slow gastric emptying, which can affect the entire digestive system

Prevention and management:

- Increase fiber gradually (fruits, vegetables, whole grains).
- Stay well-hydrated (aim for half your body weight in ounces daily).
- Regular physical activity, even just walking.
- Probiotic foods or supplements.
- Over-the-counter stool softeners, if needed.

When to worry: no bowel movement for more than three days, severe abdominal pain, or significant bloating

Fatigue: The Adjustment Period

What's normal: mild to moderate tiredness during the first two to four weeks as your body adjusts

Management strategies:

- Prioritize sleep (aim for seven to nine hours nightly).
- Light physical activity, like walking, can boost energy.
- Ensure adequate nutrition despite reduced appetite.
- Limit caffeine late in the day.
- Take short naps if needed (but not longer than 30 minutes).

When to check in: severe fatigue that interferes with work or daily activities

Other Common Side Effects

- **Heartburn or acid reflux:**
    - Eat smaller meals.
    - Avoid trigger foods (spicy, acidic, fatty).
    - Don't lie down within two to three hours after eating.
    - Consider over-the-counter antacids.
- **Headaches:**
    - Stay well-hydrated.
    - Maintain regular meal times even with reduced appetite.
    - Monitor for patterns (timing, triggers).
    - Over-the-counter pain relievers as needed.
- **Injection site reactions:**
    - Rotate injection sites.
    - Ensure medication is at room temperature.

- Clean the injection site with alcohol before injecting.
- Apply ice after injection if needed.

Side Effects Are Temporary, Benefits Are Lasting

If you're reading through this list feeling overwhelmed, take a moment to breathe. The majority of people experience only mild side effects that improve significantly within two to four weeks. Your body is remarkably good at adapting to new medications, and what feels challenging in week two often becomes barely noticeable by week six.

Most importantly, you're not expected to tough it out alone. Your healthcare provider prescribed this medication because they believe the benefits will outweigh temporary discomfort. Don't hesitate to reach out with any questions or concerns. Many side effects can be managed with simple adjustments to timing, food choices, or over-the-counter remedies. Keep perspective: The side effects are your body adjusting to positive changes. The nausea indicates that the medication is slowing your digestion and regulating your appetite. The fatigue often signals that your metabolism is resetting. These temporary inconveniences are often the pathway to lasting improvements in energy, health, and quality of life.

If side effects feel unmanageable, that's valuable information for your healthcare team, not a sign of failure. Sometimes a slower titration schedule, a different medication, or additional support strategies can make all the difference. The goal is to find an approach that works for your body and your life.

Non-Scale Victories: Redefining Success

The scale can be a liar, especially in the first 90 days. Water retention, muscle changes, hormonal fluctuations, and normal daily variations can mask real progress. That's why tracking non-scale victories (NSVs) is a game-changer for maintaining motivation and recognizing genuine improvements. Let's take a look at the different NSVs you might want to start paying attention to.

I bet there are more than you realized!

Physical NSVs

- **Clothing changes:**
  - Jeans that button more easily.
  - Belts moved to tighter notches.
  - Shirts that feel less snug across the stomach.
  - Underwear or bras that fit better.
- **Energy and stamina:**
  - Climbing stairs without getting winded.
  - Having energy for evening activities.
  - Sleeping better and waking more refreshed.
  - Less afternoon energy crashes.
- **Physical comfort:**
  - Reduced joint pain, especially knees and back.
  - Less heartburn or acid reflux.
  - Improved mobility and flexibility.
  - Fewer headaches.

Behavioral NSVs

- **Food relationship changes:**
  - Leaving food on your plate naturally.
  - Feeling satisfied with smaller portions.
  - Less obsessive thinking about food.
  - Reduced late-night snacking.
- **Social situations:**
  - Feeling comfortable at restaurants.
  - Not feeling deprived at parties or gatherings.
  - Making food choices without internal battles.
  - Enjoying meals without guilt.

- **Daily habits:**
    - Choosing to take stairs instead of elevators.
    - Parking farther away without thinking about it.
    - Preparing healthier meals at home.
    - Drinking more water throughout the day.

Emotional and Mental NSVs

- **Mood improvements:**
    - Feeling more confident in social situations.
    - Less anxiety around food choices.
    - Improved self-image and body acceptance.
    - Greater sense of control over health.
- **Mental clarity:**
    - Better focus during afternoon meetings.
    - Less brain fog after meals.
    - Improved decision-making around food.
    - Feeling more present during daily activities.

The Moment It Clicks

Six weeks into my Ozempic journey, I experienced an NSV that had nothing to do with food or the scale. I was running late for a meeting and had to park three blocks away from the office building. In the past, this would have meant arriving sweaty and out of breath, needing a few minutes to recover before I could think clearly.

But that day, I walked those three blocks at a brisk pace and climbed two flights of stairs to the meeting room without my usual huffing and puffing. I sat down and realized I felt... normal. Alert. Ready to engage. My back wasn't aching from the walk, my knees weren't protesting the stairs, and I wasn't mentally calculating how long I'd need to catch my breath.

It wasn't until later that evening that I realized what had happened. The 15 pounds I'd lost had taken significant pressure off my joints and improved my cardiovascular fitness in a way that felt effortless. I wasn't trying to exercise more or push myself harder. I was simply moving through my day with less physical resistance.

This is what I want you to watch for in your own journey. The victories might not be dramatic moments of willpower or major lifestyle overhauls. They might be climbing a flight of stairs without thinking about it, playing with your kids without your back aching, or having energy for evening activities that used to feel impossible.

These everyday moments of feeling comfortable in your body and confident in your physical capabilities are often the most meaningful indicators that something fundamental has shifted. Don't wait for perfect numbers on a scale to celebrate. These quiet improvements in how you move through the world are the real prize.

Managing Expectations and Staying Motivated

Around week four, something predictable happens to most people starting GLP-1 therapy: the initial excitement starts to fade, and reality sets in. Maybe the side effects are lingering longer than expected, or the scale isn't moving as quickly as you'd hoped. Perhaps you're seeing other people's dramatic progress online and wondering why your journey looks different.

This is the point where many people start second-guessing themselves.

- Is this working for me?
- Should I feel more dramatic changes by now?
- What if I'm one of the people this doesn't work for?

These doubts are not only normal, they're practically universal.

The truth is, our culture has conditioned us to expect instant results, especially when it comes to weight loss. We're used to seeing dramatic transformations on social media and TV shows that compress months of progress into highlight reels. But real, sustainable change happens on a different timeline, one that's often messier and more gradual than the stories we see online.

As we've learned, GLP-1 medications aren't magic bullets that work the same way for everyone. Some people see dramatic early results, others experience steady, slower progress. Some individuals lose weight quickly but struggle with side effects, while others experience gradual changes but feel amazing.

Neither path is wrong, and neither predicts your long-term success. Here, I aim to help you understand what realistic progress looks like, how to handle the inevitable moments of doubt, and most importantly, how to stay motivated when the journey doesn't unfold exactly as you expected.

What "Normal" Progress Looks Like

1. **Week 1-2:** Minimal weight loss (one to three lbs), mostly water weight. Focus on side effect management and routine building.
2. **Week 3-4:** More noticeable appetite changes. Possible three to six lbs weight loss. Early NSVs are starting to appear.
3. **Month 2:** Weight loss may average one to two lbs per week. Strong appetite suppression. Clear behavioral changes.
4. **Month 3:** Cumulative weight loss of 8-15 lbs is typical. Established routines. Noticeable improvements in energy and mood.

Always keep in mind that individual variation is huge. Some people see faster results, while others see slower ones. Factors that affect your timeline include starting weight, other medications, stress levels, sleep quality, and individual metabolism.

Overcoming Common Mental Challenges

"Is this working for me?"

This doubt usually hits around week 3-4. Look beyond the scale. Review your baseline measurements and NSV list. Often, changes are happening that the scale doesn't reflect.

"I'm not losing as fast as [person online]"

Social media and online forums can trigger comparison anxiety. Remember that people often share their best weeks or use different timelines. Focus on your own baseline and progress.

"What if I can't tolerate the side effects?"

Most side effects improve within two to four weeks. If they don't, talk to your provider about adjusting your dose or trying a different medication. Having side effects doesn't mean you're failing.

"I missed a dose/made a mistake"

Perfectionism kills progress. One missed dose, one bad meal, one off day doesn't erase your progress. Focus on getting back on track rather than self-criticism.

Building Resilience Through the Journey

- **Celebrate small wins weekly:** Write down three things that went well each week, no matter how minor they seem.
- **Connect with support:** Whether it's online communities, friends, or family members, don't try to do this alone.
- **Practice self-compassion:** Talk to yourself the way you would to a good friend going through the same experience.
- **Focus on habits, not just outcomes:** Building sustainable routines matters more than any single week's results.
- **Keep perspective:** This is a marathon, not a sprint. The habits you build in these first 90 days will serve you for years to come.

Real Stories of Overcoming Early Doubts

Maria, 51, accounting manager: "At week 6, I'd only lost four pounds and was ready to quit. My doctor reminded me to look beyond the numbers on the scale. I realized I'd been sleeping through the night for the first time in years and had energy to cook dinner instead of ordering takeout. Those changes motivated me to stick with it. By month 3, the weight loss caught up."

David, 43, construction supervisor: "The first month was rough—nausea, fatigue, and barely any weight loss. I kept thinking about the $300 I was spending each month. But then I noticed I wasn't popping Tums every night for heartburn, and I could bend over to tie my shoes without my back screaming. Those little things reminded me this was working, just not how I expected."

Lisa, 38, working mom: "I almost gave up during week 4 when I gained two pounds after a work conference. My online support group reminded me that travel, stress, and hormonal changes all affect the scale. They encouraged me to look at my overall trend, rather than focusing on my daily fluctuations. That perspective shift changed everything for me."

Progress isn't linear, and the most meaningful changes often happen gradually and quietly.

Practicing Self-Compassion During Setbacks

The voice in your head during challenging moments matters more than you might think. Instead of harsh self-criticism, try reframing setbacks with kindness:

Instead of: "I'm failing again, just like every other diet"

Try: "My body is adjusting to significant changes, and some bumps are normal."

Instead of: "I should be losing weight faster."

Try: "My body is working at its own pace, and other improvements are happening too."

Instead of: "I can't handle the side effects."

Try: "These symptoms are temporary signs that the medication is working."

Actionable Self-Compassion Tools

The Three-Minute Reset: When frustration hits, take three deep breaths and ask yourself: "What would I tell my best friend in this situation?" Offer yourself the same kindness.

Progress Jar: Write down every small victory on a piece of paper and put it in a jar. When motivation is low, take a moment to reflect on how far you've come.

Daily Affirmation Practice: Choose one phrase that resonates with you:

- "I am learning to trust my body's wisdom."

- "Every day on this medication is an investment in my future health."
- "Progress isn't always visible, but it's always happening."

The Photo Journal: Take a weekly photo in the same outfit and lighting. Often, changes are visible in photos before you notice them in the mirror. Include notes about how you felt that week, not just how you looked.

These tools help build resilience for the inevitable challenges while keeping focus on long-term health rather than short-term perfection.

Building Sustainable Routines

The first 90 days are extremely important for establishing patterns that will support your long-term success. These routines should feel manageable, not overwhelming. Below are my top tips for building sustainable, manageable routines across the different areas of this journey.

Medication Management

- **Set consistent timing:** Choose a day and time that works with your schedule and stick to it. Many people prefer weekend mornings when they're not rushed.
- **Use multiple reminders:** Phone alarms, calendar notifications, and even pill reminder apps can help until the routine becomes automatic.
- **Track adherence:** Mark successful doses on a calendar or in an app. Seeing your consistency builds confidence.
- **Plan for travel:** Know how to store and transport your medication safely. Set backup alarms in different time zones.

Meal Planning and Preparation

- **Start simple:** Focus on having healthy options available rather than complicated meal plans. Stock protein sources, vegetables, and easy-to-prepare items.

- **Batch preparation:** Spend 30-60 minutes on weekends preparing basics like washed vegetables, cooked proteins, or portioned snacks.
- **Adjust portions gradually:** As your appetite changes, use smaller plates and bowls to help portions appear more satisfying.
- **Plan for social eating:** Consider your restaurant options, potluck contributions, and party strategies in advance.

Activity and Movement

- **Start where you are:** If you're sedentary, begin with 10-minute daily walks. If you're active, maintain your current routine while your energy adjusts.
- **Track naturally:** Use your smartphone's built-in step counter or a simple fitness tracker to monitor daily movement without obsessing.
- **Build gradually:** Add 5-10 minutes of activity weekly as energy and motivation improve.
- **Find enjoyment:** Choose activities that you genuinely enjoy. Dancing, gardening, playing with pets, or walking while listening to podcasts all count.

Sleep and Stress Management

- **Prioritize sleep:** GLP-1 medications work better when you're well-rested. Aim for seven to nine hours and maintain consistent sleep/wake times.
- **Manage stress:** High stress can interfere with weight loss and increase side effects. Find simple stress-relief techniques that work for you.
- **Create buffer time:** Don't pack your schedule too tightly. Allow extra time for appointments, meal preparation, and self-care.

Routine-building isn't about perfection. Let your routine align with your actual life and try out different systems until you find one that sticks, knowing that your needs will shift as your treatment progresses (Murray et al., 2020; Polhemus et al., 2022). Soon, you'll find that the routines you set now will give you the resilience to adapt to challenges ahead, even as your medication, habits, or goals change.

Tools and Templates for Long-Term Monitoring

Weekly reflection template: Copy this into your notes app or print it out:

Week of: [Date]

Current dose: [Amount]

This week's wins:

1.
2.
3.

Challenges faced:

1.
2.

Side effects (rate 1-10):

- Nausea:
- Fatigue:
- Other:

NSVs noticed:

- Physical:
- Behavioral:
- Emotional:

Energy level (average 1-10):

Sleep quality (average 1-10):

Hunger/appetite changes:

Goals for next week:

1.

2.

Monthly Check-In Questions:

- What patterns am I noticing in my energy, mood, or eating habits?
- Which strategies have been most helpful for managing side effects?
- What aspects of my routine need adjustment?
- How can I better support my progress next month?

Preparing for Your First Follow-Up

Most providers schedule follow-up appointments four to six weeks after starting GLP-1 therapy. Being prepared helps you get the most from these visits.

What to Bring

- **Your tracking data:** Whether it's app screenshots, journal entries, or simple notes, bring evidence of your experience.
- **Questions list:** Write down questions beforehand so you don't forget them during the appointment.
- **Current medications:** Any changes since starting GLP-1 therapy.
- **Specific concerns:** Be ready to discuss side effects, effectiveness, or any problems you've experienced.

Questions to Ask

- **About progress:**
    - Are my results typical for this timeline?
    - Should we adjust my dose or stay at the current level?
    - What improvements should I focus on tracking?
- **About side effects:**
    - Are my side effects within normal range?
    - What strategies might help manage [specific side effect]?
    - When should I call if side effects worsen?
- **About the future:**
    - How long do most people stay on this medication?
    - What's our long-term plan for dose adjustments?
    - What other lifestyle changes would enhance my results?

Setting Yourself Up for Long-Term Success

The first 90 days are just the beginning of your GLP-1 journey.

The habits, routines, and mindset you develop during this period will determine your long-term success.

Key Principles for the Long Haul

- **Consistency over perfection:** It's better to be 80% consistent over months than 100% perfect for a few weeks.
- **Progress over performance:** Focus on moving forward rather than comparing yourself to others or achieving arbitrary standards.
- **Flexibility over rigidity:** Life will throw curveballs. Build adaptability into your routines rather than rigid rules.

- **Health over just weight:** Weight loss is one benefit of GLP-1 therapy, but improvements in energy, mood, sleep, and overall health are equally valuable.

Preparing for Challenges

- **Weight loss plateaus:** They're normal and temporary. Having strategies ready helps you stay the course.
- **Life disruptions:** Travel, illness, work stress, or family changes will test your routines. Plan how you'll adapt rather than abandon your efforts.
- **Side effect changes:** As doses increase or your body adjusts, new challenges may arise. Stay in communication with your healthcare team.
- **Motivation fluctuations:** Enthusiasm naturally wanes over time. Having systems in place helps you continue even when motivation is low.

These early days of your GLP-1 journey are about much more than initial weight loss. They're about learning to trust your body's new signals, building sustainable routines, and developing the mindset and habits that will support long-term success. The tracking systems you establish now, the side effect management strategies you develop, and the realistic expectations you set will serve you well beyond these initial months.

By now, you should have a clear sense of how your body responds to the medication, what side effects you may experience, and how to recognize progress in multiple forms. You've hopefully established routines for medication management, developed strategies for handling challenges, and begun to appreciate victories that go beyond the scale.

As you move beyond the adjustment period, your focus will naturally shift from managing the initial effects of GLP-1 therapy to optimizing your results through nutrition, movement, and lifestyle choices. The foundation you've built during these first three months becomes the platform for deeper changes in how you fuel your body, stay active, and maintain the improvements you've gained.

The next chapter will guide you through the practical aspects of eating well on GLP-1s, helping you navigate the unique nutritional considerations that come with reduced appetite and altered hunger cues. You'll learn how to ensure you're getting adequate nutrition despite eating less, how to navigate social eating situations, and how to build meal patterns that support both your medication's effectiveness and your long-term health goals.

Chapter 7:

Life Gets Lighter: The Everyday Victories of GLP-1s

Two months into my Ozempic journey, I had a moment that had nothing to do with weight loss. I was helping my partner move furniture, something that would have left me in agony for days before. But that evening, my back felt... fine. Not perfect, but manageable. Normal. I realized I'd been so focused on the scale that I'd almost missed this massive victory: I was moving through life with less pain.

In the previous chapter, we touched on non-scale victories as part of tracking your progress during the first 90 days. You learned to recognize early signs, such as improved sleep, reduced cravings, or fitting into clothes more comfortably. Now we're going to dive deeper into why these victories matter so much for long-term success, how to systematically track them, and most importantly, how to use them as your primary source of motivation when the scale isn't cooperating.

This chapter is about making NSVs central to your journey rather than just a side note. The truth is that sustainable motivation doesn't come from watching numbers drop. It comes from feeling the difference in your body, your energy, and your relationship with food and movement.

Why Non-Scale Victories Matter

For many on a weight-loss journey, progress is measured in numbers, especially the one on the bathroom scale. Yet as research on well-being deepens, those invested in true transformation begin to notice that the scale can't tell the full story. NSVs are the daily triumphs, small or large, that mark deeper shifts—transformations that bring real joy, freedom, and energy back to everyday life (*Non Scale Victories*, n.d.; *Keeping Track of Your Success*, 2022).

NSVs represent more than fleeting moments of achievement. They're all-around improvements in how you feel, move, and interact with the world. Imagine taking the stairs after a work meeting and realizing how little it takes out of you. Perhaps you notice a fuller breath at the top, or that normal knee twinge simply doesn't appear. These sorts of victories build up, creating lasting motivation that persists even through plateaus and setbacks.

The Problem With Scale-Only Focus

When you only track weight, you miss important information about your health journey. The scale can't measure

- energy levels that let you play with your kids after work.
- joint pain that's disappeared or significantly reduced.
- sleep quality that leaves you refreshed instead of groggy.
- mental clarity that carries you through afternoon meetings.
- confidence that lets you say yes to social invitations.

Worse, focusing only on the scale can sabotage motivation during normal fluctuations. Water retention, hormonal changes, muscle development, and even what you ate yesterday can all affect the number you see, creating unnecessary stress and disappointment.

What Research Shows

Studies consistently show that people who track multiple health markers beyond weight tend to have better long-term success (Hosseini et al., 2023; Lau et al., 2022). Improvements in blood pressure, cholesterol, A1C, and inflammatory markers indicate positive changes within your body, even when the scale remains stubborn. According to the American Diabetes Association, reducing A1C by even one percentage point can lower the risk of diabetes complications by up to 37%, representing a substantial shift in long-term well-being (Riddle et al., 2018). For many midlife professionals whose lives already demand constant mental energy, relief from food obsession can feel life-changing. Less time spent thinking about the next meal, planning around cravings, or mentally wrestling with hunger means more energy for work, relationships, and activities that bring joy. What's striking is how these victories quietly shift mindsets. Confidence grows stronger.

With every walk taken and every balanced meal chosen, self-doubt and guilt get pushed aside, making room for self-compassion and personal growth. It becomes possible to weather the inevitable plateaus or setbacks, knowing they don't erase the benefits already felt.

Imagine coming home after a packed day, setting down the keys, and realizing you have more than enough energy to talk with family, whip up a meal, or even sit with a book. The victories here show up in laughter shared, moments seized, and tiredness replaced by a sense of hope. These are the wins that motivate continued effort, refocus attention away from fleeting numbers, and set the stage for the honest, lasting outcomes that matter most for people living full, demanding lives. As NSVs become more visible, they pave the way for fresh stories. Stories of rediscovered strength, bolder social choices, and proof that change is possible at every stage.

Real-Life Non-Scale Victories

Health Improvements You Can Measure

Tina's Blood Pressure Victory

Tina used to hold her breath during every doctor's appointment when it was time for her blood pressure check. Last spring, at her annual visit, her doctor smiled. Her readings had dropped into the healthy range, making it possible to consider lowering her medication. For Tina, that brought a rush of relief and pride. Better blood pressure meant she felt safer leaving the house alone, had steadier energy at work, and could laugh with her daughter without worrying about chest tightness.

Tiffany's Lab Work Surprise

Tiffany, a 52-year-old nurse, noticed something unexpected at her annual physical. "My doctor reviewed my labs and said, 'Whatever you're doing, keep doing it.' My cholesterol had dropped 40 points, my triglycerides were down, and my liver enzymes had normalized. I'd been so focused on losing weight that I forgot GLP-1s were also protecting my heart and metabolic health."

For people on a GLP-1 journey, stories like Tina and Jennifer's pop up everywhere. They reinforce what research shows: improving cardiovascular health gives back not only physical freedom but also a sense of peace of mind that spills into daily routines (Turabi et al., 2025). Blood pressure and cholesterol are tied to future health risks, but today, they also affect your energy levels for family, travel, and the things you love.

Energy and Stamina Changes

Marcus's Mobility Transformation

A few months after starting GLP-1 therapy, Marcus noticed a difference in his mornings. The flight of stairs from his bedroom no longer left him winded. He noticed he could keep walking while chatting on the phone, without needing frequent breaks. Then, when vacationing with friends, he realized he'd trekked five miles through city streets, all without back pain or lagging behind.

These moments were small but meaningful: dog walks doubled, garden projects finished in a weekend, sprints to catch the train were possible without dread. Studies show that lifestyle changes, including medication and regular physical activity, lead to increased energy, improved stamina, and changes in body composition (Niezgoda et al., 2025). Many users are startled to realize their limits keep shifting outward, offering fresh reasons to keep moving and stay connected to their goals.

Relationship With Food

Maya's Restaurant Revelation

Maya spent years sizing up restaurant menus with nervous calculation. Calories haunted her, and every plate felt like a test she had to pass or fail. GLP-1 support worked in the background. One night, she noticed she had left food on her plate and didn't feel compelled to finish it. Instead of guilt, she felt oddly free. She enjoyed her meal, chatted with her partner, and savored a dessert without anxiety.

This shift is real for countless GLP-1 users who report feeling full faster, being less drawn to second helpings, and being better able to listen to hunger cues rather than following old patterns (Turabi et al., 2025). What grows alongside satisfaction is a new ease at meals: conversations flow, focus shifts from restriction to enjoyment, and shame starts to fall away. No calorie app can measure the freedom that comes from simply being present at a table, or from breaking the habit of calling foods "good" or "bad."

Social and Confidence Wins

Charmaine's Confidence Breakthrough

On a sunny afternoon, Charmaine put on her favorite red jacket, the one she'd bought years ago on a hopeful shopping trip but never wore. It fit, and just right. That night, at her cousin's wedding, she didn't hide from the camera. She laughed for real in family pictures. At work, she volunteered to present at an event, something she'd avoided when self-consciousness made her shrink.

David's Family Gathering

David's victory came at a family gathering. "For years, I dreaded events with extended family because I knew there'd be comments about my weight or 'helpful' diet advice. At my nephew's graduation party, I realized halfway through that I'd been enjoying conversations, not thinking about food or feeling self-conscious. That mental freedom was worth more than any number on the scale."

Many GLP-1 users describe moments like these: stepping out with confidence, tackling social invitations that used to cause worry, and taking on activities without holding back. Each event attended, each piece of clothing rediscovered, each connection strengthened, offers validation. Self-respect grows, and real confidence has space to breathe.

It can be easy to overlook these gains when the scale isn't moving fast or when setbacks appear. Yet the thread running through every one of these stories is simple: Wins that aren't measured in pounds build motivation from the inside out. When you open your eyes to them, even the small shifts, like a regular morning walk, a shared family meal, or the courage to say yes, carry energy. Noticing these improvements can become a habit in its own right. By learning to track and name each victory, you loosen the grip of old expectations and make space for lasting change. Steps, smiles, and shared moments are a new kind of progress that show up, ready to be counted, showing day by day that life really does get lighter.

Tracking and Celebrating Your Non-Scale Victories

It's easy to laser-focus on the scale when tracking progress with GLP-1 medications, but there's a whole world of NSVs that bring motivation and true satisfaction. To make NSVs really count, tracking them is important. Setting up a dedicated weekly or monthly NSV checklist transforms fleeting moments into a gallery of progress.

Try these practical steps to get started:

1. Set up a checklist in your preferred app, such as MyFitnessPal, Apple Health, or a simple digital journal.
2. Fill your tracker with prompts such as:
    - "Today I walked up two flights of stairs with no pain."
    - "I said no to a snack because I wasn't really hungry."
    - "I enjoyed dinner at a restaurant without worrying about calories."
3. Capture these wins as they happen: take a quick picture, record a digital badge, or write a one-sentence note.
4. Save photos or entries in a folder, even a collection as simple as "Small Wins 2025" on your phone, can work.
5. Use push notifications or calendar reminders with prompts like "What NSV did I achieve today?" or "Celebrate a win tonight."

Use this simple weekly NSV journal:

This Week's Energy Wins:

- Morning energy level (1-10):
- Afternoon slump? (Yes/No):
- Evening activities I had energy for:

This Week's Physical Wins:

- Activities that felt easier:
- Pain levels compared to last month:
- Movement milestones (stairs, distance, etc.):

This Week's Food Relationship Wins:

- Times I ate until satisfied, not stuffed:
- Social eating situations handled well:
- Cravings that were easier to manage:

This Week's Confidence Wins:

- Social situations I felt comfortable in:
- Clothes that fit better:
- Compliments or comments received:

This Week's Overall Victory:

- What I'm most proud of this week:

Digital Tools and Apps

Apps and digital tools work well for habit-driven, goal-oriented individuals. Consider making use of the following:

- **MyFitnessPal or Apple Health:** Create custom tracking categories for NSVs alongside traditional metrics.
- **Habit tracking apps:** Mark daily victories like "walked without pain" or "enjoyed a meal without guilt."
- **Photo documentation:** Take weekly progress photos in the same outfit and lighting—changes often show up visually before numerically.

- **Notes app victories:** Keep a running list titled "Small Wins 2025" and add to it whenever something positive happens.
- **Push notifications:** Set reminders that prompt "What NSV did I achieve today?" or "Celebrate a win tonight."

Journaling Prompts for Reflection

If you prefer to journal, whether that be by hand or digitally, you can use these prompts to help identify NSVs you might be overlooking:

Weekly reflection:

- What felt easier this week compared to a month ago?
- What did my body allow me to do that would have been harder before?
- What food-related moment am I most proud of?
- What physical discomfort has improved or disappeared?

During challenging weeks:

- Even though the scale didn't move, what else improved?
- What non-weight victory can I celebrate right now?
- How is my life different today than before starting GLP-1s?
- What activity or situation feels more manageable now?

Sharing Your Victories

Sharing these moments with a community adds another layer of support. Many people these days are active on wellness forums, Reddit groups, or group texts. Posting about your everyday wins can bring you a wealth of encouragement and accountability. Try sharing before/after energy levels, reframed setbacks, or new routines in these digital spaces. A quick photo captioned, "Walked the block with no breaks!" or a comment about resisting old habits can draw cheers from others. Celebrating friends' NSVs works both ways, so be sure to uplift others while you're there, too. The mutual uplift creates a ripple effect, keeping everyone involved motivated.

Using NSVs to Navigate Plateaus and Setbacks

No health journey is perfectly linear. There are weeks when jeans feel tight again, or progress on the scale seems stuck. That's when NSVs have the most power. Week 8 personally hit me hard. The scale hadn't moved in two weeks despite consistent medication, a reasonable diet, and regular movement. I felt the old familiar frustration creeping in, the voice saying, "This isn't working," and "You're wasting your time."

That's when I pulled out my NSV list. In those same two weeks where the scale stayed put, I'd walked three miles without my back flaring up, slept through the night consistently, and noticed my afternoon brain fog had disappeared. My body was changing even when the scale wasn't.

The Power of Reframing

Plateaus are inevitable on any health journey. Your body needs time to adjust, recalibrate, and consolidate changes. Redirecting focus is key here: When frustration kicks in, check your NSV list and reframe what you're experiencing.

Instead of: "Nothing's working, I've been stuck for two weeks."

Reframe as: "My weight is stabilizing while other improvements continue. What non-scale changes have I noticed?"

Instead of: "I must be doing something wrong."

Reframe as: "My body is adjusting. What's going well that I can build on?"

Instead of: "I should just give up."

Reframe as: "This pause doesn't erase my progress. What victories can I celebrate today?"

Progress, Not Perfection

The ultimate goal is forward movement, even when that movement isn't visible on a scale. Some weeks, you'll notice improvements in energy. Other weeks, it's about reduced pain or better sleep.

Still others might bring social confidence or food freedom.

Tips for staying motivated through plateaus:

- Review your NSV list weekly, especially when the scale isn't moving.
- Set goals unrelated to weight (walk a certain distance, try a new activity, improve sleep quality).
- Connect with your support community about non-scale progress.
- Remember that metabolic changes can take time to translate into weight loss.
- Take progress photos monthly—changes often show up visually before numerically.

Learning From Setbacks

Even setbacks contain valuable information. Maybe a week of poor sleep led to increased cravings. Perhaps stress affected your appetite control. These aren't failures—they're data points that help you understand your body better.

When facing setbacks:

- Look for patterns in your NSV tracking.
- Identify which victories remained stable even during challenges.
- Recognize that some progress continues even when other areas struggle.
- Use NSVs as evidence that you haven't lost everything during a difficult period.

Celebrating Your Victories

Collecting small wins shifts the focus from perfection to progress. Each NSV, tracked and celebrated, adds up, building your confidence, encouraging pride, and deepening self-care. Celebration doesn't have to be elaborate. Sometimes it's as simple as acknowledging a win in your journal or sharing it with a friend. The key is making celebration a habit, not something you only do after major milestones.

Small Ways to Celebrate

- **Daily acknowledgments:** End each day by naming one victory, no matter how small.
- **Victory jar:** Write down NSVs on slips of paper and collect them in a jar to read during tough weeks.
- **Sharing with accountability partners:** Text or message someone when you notice a victory.
- **Progress photos:** Take a photo when you notice a physical NSV and keep them in a dedicated album.
- **Treating yourself:** Reward NSVs with non-food treats—new workout gear, a massage, or a book you've been wanting.
- **Social media shares:** Post about victories in supportive online communities where others will celebrate with you.

Making It Sustainable

The habit of noticing and celebrating NSVs becomes more valuable the longer you practice it. Over time, you'll train yourself to see progress in multiple dimensions rather than fixating on a single number. This mindset shift is what separates short-term dieting from lasting transformation. The bigger story isn't just about pounds lost but also about the strength gained in daily living and joy found in new routines.

Moving Forward With NSV Awareness

Understanding and tracking non-scale victories transforms your relationship with health and wellness. Instead of deriving all your motivation from external measurements, you learn to recognize internal changes that often matter more for quality of life.

As you continue your GLP-1 journey, keep these principles in mind:

- **NSVs are diverse:** They show up in physical health, mental clarity, emotional well-being, social confidence, and daily capabilities.

- **NSVs are personal:** What matters to you might not matter to someone else, and that's perfectly fine.
- **NSVs are cumulative:** Small victories build on each other, creating sustainable momentum.
- **NSVs are resilient:** They can persist even during plateaus or setbacks, providing stable motivation.

This broader view of success helps you stay confident through ups and downs, reminding you that progress is about feeling stronger, more energetic, and more connected to life. Let these victories guide your journey, bringing steady momentum and joy that extends far beyond any single measurement on a scale.

The next chapter will explore practical nutrition strategies that complement your GLP-1 medication, helping you fuel your body appropriately while working with your changed appetite and hunger cues.

Chapter 8:

Smart Nutrition: The GLP-1 Meal Blueprint

Your appetite has changed. Meals that used to disappear in minutes now sit half-finished on your plate. The constant hunger that drove your day has quieted down to occasional whispers. This shift raises new questions: How do you eat enough when you're rarely hungry? What should you prioritize when every bite counts? How do you build meal routines that work with your new biology instead of fighting against it?

This chapter answers those questions with practical strategies you can use starting today. We'll cover how to prevent undereating while honoring your reduced appetite, why protein becomes your nutritional anchor, and how to build simple meal patterns that require minimal time and mental energy. You'll also get my actual breakfast rotation, the seven-day cycle that's kept me on track for years, and learn how to adapt these principles to restaurants, social events, and the unpredictable reality of busy life.

Appetite Drop: Understanding Appetite Changes

The first thing you notice on GLP-1s is how fast fullness arrives. Two bites into lunch and you're done. A half-sandwich sits wrapped on your desk. Dinner leftovers pile up in the fridge. If you've spent years finishing every plate or battling constant hunger, this new reality can feel disorienting. Your appetite signals have fundamentally changed because GLP-1 medications work on both your brain and your gut, telling your body it's satisfied sooner and slowing stomach emptying. What used to be a gradual build of hunger now feels like an on-off switch.

You might forget to eat entirely when you're focused on work, then realize hours have passed without a single hunger pang. Instead of seeing this as a problem to fix, think of it as your new normal, and learn to work with it rather than against it, as that makes all the difference.

Nutrient Density Over Volume

When your portions shrink, every bite needs to work harder. This is where nutrient density becomes your best friend. Instead of thinking about how much you can eat, focus on packing maximum nutrition in smaller portions.

A cup of Greek yogurt with chia seeds delivers more protein, healthy fats, and fiber than a bagel twice its size. A few soft-boiled eggs with avocado slices give you sustained energy that a muffin never could. A handful of walnuts over leafy greens brings vitamins, minerals, and good fats in a small package.

The goal isn't to eat less for the sake of eating less. It's to make sure what you do eat fuels your body properly. When you only have room for half your usual portion, that half needs to count.

Preventing Undereating Without Forcing Food

With hunger signals muted, it's easy to accidentally undereat. You might go all morning without thinking about food, work through lunch, and suddenly find yourself exhausted at 3 p.m. with no clear reason why.

Low energy, brain fog, irritability, dizziness, these are your body's way of saying it needs fuel, even when traditional hunger signals aren't firing. The solution isn't to force yourself to eat when you're full. It's to build a basic structure that ensures you're getting enough throughout the day. Set a minimum: at least three meals or substantial snacks daily, regardless of hunger. Use phone reminders if needed. Keep portable options ready: protein bars in your bag, string cheese in the office fridge, almonds in your desk drawer.

When the reminder goes off, check in with your body. Even if you're not hungry, a small protein-rich snack can prevent that afternoon crash.

Learning Your New Hunger Cues

Your body is still sending signals; they're just quieter now. A slight pressure in your stomach. Losing interest in the food on your plate. Feeling ready to focus on conversation instead of eating. These subtle cues replace the loud, insistent hunger you might be used to.

Practice the pause: set your fork down halfway through meals and check in. Are you still hungry, or are you eating from habit? There's a difference between "not full" and "still hungry," and GLP-1s help you find that middle ground.

Some people find it helpful to use a simple 1-10 hunger scale in a journal. A 1 is starving, 10 is uncomfortably stuffed, and 5-6 is satisfied. Eating when you're at a 3-4 and stopping at a 6-7 keeps energy steady without overeating or undereating. It sounds mechanical at first, but after a few weeks, it becomes intuitive (Mozaffarian et al., 2025).

Flexible meal timing also helps. If three large meals feel like too much, try five smaller ones. If breakfast doesn't appeal until mid-morning, adjust your schedule. The rigid breakfast-lunch-dinner structure might not fit your new appetite patterns, and that's completely fine.

Meal planning on GLP-1s is all about fit: making your nutrition suit your new fullness signals and your real life. The next step involves dialing in the protein and nutrient balance in every meal, making sure smaller portions work as hard as possible for strength, energy, and satiety.

Protein Power: Essential Nutritional Needs

When portions shrink, protein becomes your nutritional anchor. It preserves muscle during weight loss, stabilizes blood sugar levels, keeps you fuller longer, and gives your body the building blocks it needs to function well. For most adults on GLP-1s, a good target is 1.0 to 1.2 grams of protein per kilogram of body weight per day. If you weigh 160 pounds (roughly 73 kg), aim for 75 to 88 grams of protein each day. Breaking that down into meals, you're looking at about 20 to 30 grams per meal (Lonnie et al., 2018; Mamerow et al., 2014).

This isn't arbitrary. Research shows that spreading protein evenly throughout the day, rather than loading it all at dinner, better supports muscle maintenance and gives you more sustained energy (Mamerow et al., 2014). Your body can only use so much protein at once for muscle building, about 30 grams per meal for most people. After that, there's no added benefit.

Why Protein Matters Even More Now

During weight loss, your body can break down both muscle and fat if it doesn't get enough protein. For women in midlife, especially, preserving muscle matters. Metabolism naturally slows with age, and muscle loss accelerates that decline. Protein helps counteract both.

But protein does more than protect muscle. It stabilizes blood sugar, preventing the energy crashes that can lead to cravings. It keeps you satisfied longer, which matters when medication already reduces your appetite. And it supports bone health during periods of calorie reduction (Mamerow et al., 2014).

Easy-to-Digest Protein Sources

With reduced appetite and sometimes sensitive digestion on GLP-1s, gentle protein sources work best:

Animal-based options:

- soft scrambled eggs
- plain Greek yogurt
- cottage cheese
- poached or baked fish
- shredded chicken or turkey
- protein shakes (whey or egg white based)
- individual cheese portions

Plant-based choices:

- silken or firm tofu
- tempeh
- lentil soup

- smooth hummus
- nut butters (almond, peanut, cashew)
- pea or soy protein powders

These options are easy on your stomach and slip naturally into most meals. If you avoid animal products, focus on soy-based proteins, lentils, and pea protein, as they better match the muscle-building effects of animal sources than other plant proteins (Lonnie et al., 2018).

Spreading Protein Throughout the Day

Small, frequent servings beat one protein-heavy meal. Your body processes and uses protein more effectively when it's spread out. This also keeps energy and hunger more stable (Mamerow et al., 2014). Quick protein add-ins for busy days:

- Mix chia seeds or hemp hearts into Greek yogurt or cottage cheese.
- Top salads with shredded rotisserie chicken or cooked salmon.
- Pair fruit with nuts or individual cheese rounds.
- Tuck a hard-boiled egg, mini tuna pouch, or turkey slices into a work bag for a portable mid-afternoon snack.
- Blend up a smoothie using Greek yogurt, protein powder, spinach, and berries for a breakfast-on-the-run.

The key is making protein automatic, not something you have to think about. When it's part of every meal and snack, hitting your targets becomes effortless.

Avoiding Taste Fatigue

Eating the same protein every day gets boring fast. Rotate your choices. Use different preparations.

Change up the flavors. Eggs can be scrambled, poached, hard-boiled, or baked into frittatas. Chicken works grilled, roasted, shredded into soup, or tossed with different sauces. Greek yogurt takes on completely different characters with cinnamon and berries versus savory herbs and cucumber.

Prep a batch of baked tofu cubes on Sunday, then toss them with different stir-fry sauces throughout the week. Rotate fresh herbs like dill, basil, or chives into egg or cottage cheese dishes. Small changes prevent the monotony that makes people abandon their nutrition plans.

With a handful of tweaked routines and choices, building protein into every meal and snack becomes second nature, setting the stage for the next step: preparing these meals quickly and simply when minutes count most (Lonnie et al., 2018; Mamerow et al., 2014).

The GLP-1 Meal Blueprint: My Breakfast Rotation

Let me tell you about the routine that's kept me on track for since using GLP-1 medication. I don't follow complicated recipes or spend hours in the kitchen. I rotate through seven simple breakfast options and aim for 25-30 grams of protein for each meal.

Day 1: Eggs (Two to Three)

High protein, prepared however I feel like it that morning. Scrambled, over easy, poached—it doesn't matter. Sometimes with a bit of cheese or spinach mixed in.

Day 2: Greek Yogurt Bowl

Use plain Greek yogurt as the base. Pre-soak chia seeds for about 10 minutes (they expand and get less crunchy), then add hemp hearts, chopped walnuts, and fresh fruit. If I want it sweeter, a small drizzle of maple syrup. This one's my favorite for mornings when I'm not that hungry but know I need to eat.

Day 3: Oatmeal With Eggs

This sounds weird until you try it. I make my oatmeal normally, then in the last few minutes of cooking, I stir in a beaten egg or two. It adds protein without changing the taste much, and the texture stays creamy. It's like a warm, comforting protein boost.

Day 4: Eggs (Different Style)

Back to eggs, but prepared differently from Day 1. Maybe a frittata with vegetables, maybe hard-boiled if I'm taking breakfast on the go.

Day 5: Yogurt

Another yogurt day, sometimes switching up the toppings depending on what's in season or what I'm craving.

Day 6: Cottage Cheese Toast

2 Pieces of Toast, 3 Table spoons Cottage cheese, season with dash of honey and chili flakes.

Day 7: Protein Pancakes

This is just mashed banana mixed with eggs, and a scooop of protein powder, then cooked like pancakes. Nothing else is needed. It sounds too simple to work, but it's genuinely good, slightly sweet from the banana, and high in protein from the eggs. Perfect for a weekend morning when I want something that feels like a treat but still hits my nutritional targets.

This rotation takes the decision-making out of breakfast. I know exactly what I'm having each day, I can prep ingredients in advance, and I never get bored because it's constantly changing. More importantly, every single option delivers the protein I need to start my day strong.

You don't have to copy my exact routine. The principle is what matters: find a handful of protein-rich options you actually like, rotate them on a predictable schedule, and make breakfast automatic rather than a daily decision.

Quick Meal Planning for the Time-Starved

Building on that breakfast foundation, let's talk about making all your meals work with minimal time and mental energy. You don't need to reinvent your menu every week. In fact, that's exactly what you shouldn't do.

The 10-Minute Meal Framework

Start with shortcut ingredients. Rotisserie chicken from the grocery store becomes the protein base for salads, wraps, bowls, or stuffed peppers. Pre-washed greens, cherry tomatoes, and bottled vinaigrette turn that into a complete meal in five minutes. Add a microwaveable pouch of quinoa for more substance. Hard-boiled eggs (buy them already cooked if you want), baby carrots, and hummus make a high-protein snack or mini-meal that requires zero preparation. Canned tuna or salmon, bean pouches, and ready-made lentil salads fill in when you need something fast.

Batch cooking on weekends multiplies your options. Grill extra chicken thighs, salmon fillets, or tofu planks. Store them in portioned containers. Now you have protein ready to toss into wraps, over sweet potatoes, or into salads all week long.

When you need convenient options that align with smaller appetites and high-protein needs, look for protein bars with at least 15-20 grams of protein and minimal added sugars: brands like RXBAR, Quest, or ONE bars work well. For shakes, premade options like Fairlife Core Power, Orgain, or simple protein powder mixed with milk give you 20-30 grams of protein in seconds. Microwavable grains like quinoa pouches, brown rice cups, or farro packets from brands like Seeds of Change or Minute Rice provide quick, portion-controlled bases for bowls when paired with your prepped protein and vegetables.

For breakfast beyond my rotation, overnight oats with protein powder, cottage cheese with nuts and berries, or a protein smoothie all come together in under five minutes.

The Two-Week Meal Template

Instead of planning every meal from scratch, create a template that rotates. Pick three or four breakfast options for week one, then three or four different ones for week two. Same with lunches. Dinners stay more flexible based on what's fresh or what you're craving, but even those can follow patterns.

Week one lunches might be grilled chicken salads, tuna and white bean bowls, and veggie-packed soups. Week two cycles to grain salads, lentil wraps, and chicken lettuce cups. You're not eating the same thing every day, but you're also not inventing new meals constantly. This template approach means you can keep a standard grocery list, order online for pickup or delivery, and avoid the daily question: "What should I eat?" Decision fatigue is real, especially for busy professionals. Removing that daily choice frees up mental energy for what actually matters.

Sample Day of Eating

Here's what a typical day might look like with a smaller appetite:

- **Breakfast:** two eggs scrambled with spinach, a small handful of berries, coffee or tea
- **Lunch:** cup of lentil soup, half a whole grain pita with turkey, sliced cucumber on the side
- **Dinner:** small roasted sweet potato, palm-sized piece of grilled salmon, green salad with olive oil and avocado
- **Snacks (as needed):** slice of cheese with cherry tomatoes, mini container of cottage cheese with a few walnuts, or a protein bar

Notice the portions. Small plates work better than dinner plates. Proteins are palm-sized. Half the plate is vegetables. These visual cues make portioning automatic without measuring or calculating. If you want more variety, here are a few more sample days that work with reduced appetite:

Day 2:

- **Breakfast:** Greek yogurt bowl with chia seeds, hemp hearts, walnuts, and berries
- **Lunch:** half turkey sandwich on whole grain with side salad
- **Dinner:** baked chicken thigh with roasted Brussels sprouts and a small portion of quinoa
- **Snacks:** hard-boiled egg, handful of almonds

Day 3:

- **Breakfast:** oatmeal with eggs stirred in, topped with sliced banana
- **Lunch:** lentil soup with whole grain crackers and cucumber slices
- **Dinner:** grilled tofu with stir-fried vegetables over cauliflower rice
- **Snacks:** cottage cheese with cherry tomatoes, protein bar

Notice how these patterns repeat: protein-centered meals, vegetables taking up half the plate, small portions of quality carbohydrates, and protein-rich snacks bridging the gaps. Once you internalize these patterns, building meals becomes automatic.

Smart Snacking Strategies

Keep grab-and-go options visible and accessible. When hunger is low, you're less likely to seek out food. Having it ready increases the chances you'll actually eat when you need to. Stock your fridge, bag, and desk with:

- hard-boiled eggs
- string cheese
- roasted chickpeas
- small containers of Greek yogurt
- protein bars that actually taste good
- nut butter packets
- trail mix in portion-sized bags

These bridge the gaps between meals without requiring thought or preparation. That's exactly what you need on GLP-1s when hunger won't always remind you to eat.

Eating Out and Social Events: Staying on Track

Strong home routines make restaurant meals and social events less stressful. You're not starting from zero; you already know what works for your body. Now you're just applying those same principles in different settings.

Restaurant Strategies

Scan the menu first for protein-centered dishes. Grilled chicken, salmon, shrimp, tofu, and steak. Look for what's baked, roasted, or grilled rather than fried or breaded. Then check the sides. Most restaurants will swap fries for extra vegetables or a salad if you ask.

Don't be shy about customizing. Ask for sauce on the side. Request half portions when available. Get a takeout box when your food arrives and pack half before you start eating.

Restaurant portions are typically double what you need now, and boxing half immediately removes the temptation to keep eating past fullness.

At Italian restaurants, skip the pasta mains and look for grilled fish or chicken with vegetables. At steakhouses, the classic protein-and-vegetable pairing is always available. At sushi spots, sashimi or light nigiri gives you lean protein without excess starch.

One helpful approach: don't arrive overly hungry. Have a small protein snack before you go. It takes the edge off and makes it easier to order based on what you need rather than what looks good when you're starving.

Navigating Social Pressure

Eating with others brings its own challenges. Well-meaning friends or family might push you to eat more, try their dish, have seconds, or split dessert. You need polite but firm scripts ready.

"Everything looks amazing, but I'm actually satisfied, thank you."

"I'm saving room for the main dish."

"That looks delicious, I'll just try a bite." (Then actually just try a bite and move on.)

The "taste but don't finish" approach works at parties and buffets. Take small portions of things you're curious about, savor a few bites, then set it aside and focus on conversation. Research shows people often mirror the eating habits of those around them, so your mindful choices might actually help others, too.

Celebrations Without Guilt

Special occasions call for flexibility, not restriction. Decide ahead of time on one treat you'll truly enjoy, savor it mindfully, then focus on the non-food parts of the event. The laughter, the music, the connections with people you care about.

Bring a dish you can feel good about eating, a baked egg frittata, a substantial salad, or a Greek yogurt dip with vegetables. This guarantees you have at least one option that aligns with your goals.

Your social survival kit for any event:

- sparkling water with lime (keeps your hands busy, helps you decline extras)
- small protein snack eaten before you go (prevents arriving overly hungry)
- mental reset phrase ready ("I'm there for the people, not just the food")
- visual memory of your usual plate portions (helps you build your plate around protein and vegetables even in new places)

These strategies work at everything from work conferences to family holidays. They work because they're simple, social eating stays enjoyable, and you never feel deprived or like you're on some restrictive plan. You're just making choices that align with how your body works now.

Your Social Survival Kit

Having a few portable tools on hand prepares you for almost any occasion. Here's what to include:

- a bottle of sparkling water with lime or lemon, to sip and curb hunger before food arrives

- a small protein-rich snack, like a cheese stick or roasted chickpeas, to eat right before the event if meals are delayed
- your favorite "reset phrase," rehearsed before you go, ready to use if friends or colleagues push you to indulge: "No thanks, I had a big lunch," or "I'm pacing myself tonight."
- visual reminders of your usual plate at home, to help build your meal around protein and veggies, even in new places

By blending these strategies with your homegrown habits, you reinforce daily confidence while enjoying the connection, celebration, and surprise of eating with others.

With each outing, your choices become easier, more natural, and less likely to stray from the nutrition blueprint that supports your progress and well-being.

Building Habits That Last

The goal of all this isn't perfection. It's building a system that works with your life, your appetite, your schedule, and your preferences. My breakfast rotation works for me because it's simple, affordable, and I genuinely like all seven options.

Your rotation might look completely different.

The principles stay the same:

- prioritize protein at every meal
- pack maximum nutrition into smaller portions
- build routines that remove daily decisions
- keep convenient options always available
- adapt these strategies to restaurants and social situations
- focus on how you feel, not arbitrary rules

Your body is giving you new signals through these medications. Learning to listen and respond appropriately takes time. Be patient with yourself during the adjustment. Some days you'll nail it. Other days, you'll realize at 4 p.m. that you forgot to eat lunch. Both are normal parts of the learning process.

What matters is the overall pattern, not any single meal or day. Consistency over time builds the habits that become automatic. And when eating well feels automatic rather than effortful, that's when lasting change becomes possible.

In the next chapter, we'll look at movement, energy, and the one thing every GLP-1 user needs to know about protecting muscle while the weight comes off.

For now, focus on building your nutrition foundation, finding your rhythm with meals and snacks that work for your appetite and schedule, and trusting your body's new signals about hunger and fullness. You're not fighting your biology anymore. You're finally working with it. That shift makes all the difference.

Chapter 9:

Staying Strong: Fitness, Energy, and Protecting Muscle

Living with chronic pain, some days can be incredibly tough. On my worst days, even the thought of moving felt impossible. For a long time, that kept me stuck in the "all-or-nothing" trap: If I couldn't push hard, I wouldn't move at all. But what changed everything for me was knowing I had a medication in my system that was still working, even on the days I couldn't walk much.

That took a huge amount of pressure and stress off my shoulders.

Exercise is absolutely key, but it doesn't have to look the same for everyone, and it doesn't have to happen every single day. When the pain flared, I gave myself grace. When the weight started to come off, even small movements became easier.

That's one of the catch-22s of weight loss: Less weight makes movement easier, and more movement boosts your energy, your mood, and your results. Over time, I learned that energy doesn't just show up on its own; it comes from stacking the right habits together: eating well, carrying less weight, moving when I can, and getting decent sleep.

For me, that combination became the sweet spot. Not perfection. Not all-or-nothing. Just consistency, where and when I could find it. And the more I leaned into that, the more energy I discovered was waiting for me on the other side.

This chapter will help you find your own combination.

Finding Your Sweet Spot With GLP-1s

After years of moving through days weighed down by pain and fatigue, that first moment of relief can catch you completely off guard. Maybe it's climbing a flight of stairs without stopping halfway. Maybe it's getting out of bed without that familiar wince. For me, it was realizing I'd walked through the grocery store without constantly looking for a place to sit down. These small victories signal something bigger: your body is ready to move again.

For many people on GLP-1 medications, the changes come gradually but unmistakably. Joint pain eases. Those chronic "micro-pains" that used to follow you on errands, commutes, and even leisure walks are starting to loosen their grip (Mulcahy et al., 2025). Suddenly, daily movement feels lighter, easier, and maybe even tempting. As weight decreases and inflammation calms down, people experience real improvements in mobility and reduced pain. Even modest weight loss can significantly improve joint function and metabolic health, especially when combined with regular movement. (*The Importance of Weight Management*, 2025)

This is where things get interesting because movement itself creates a positive feedback loop. A brief walk or gentle stretching session doesn't just provide physical benefits; it genuinely lifts your mood. Studies show that moderate activity improves outlook and is associated with reduced pain, better blood sugar control, and greater overall function (Mulcahy et al., 2025; Fitch et al., 2025). That grocery store trip or walk around the block becomes "free" exercise, helping your body make the most of your medication while reinforcing all the healthy changes you're working on.

Finding Your Energy Window

Everyone has their own rhythm during the day. Maybe you wake up ready to tackle the world, but fade by noon. Maybe you're the opposite and hit your stride around lunchtime. I learned that my energy peaked mid-morning, usually an hour or two after breakfast.

That became my window for movement, even if it was just ten minutes. One of my neighbors, Justine, discovered her energy window was right after her lunch meeting. She started taking a quick walk around her office building before diving into afternoon emails. Another friend realized his evening dog walk, something he'd always seen as a chore, actually gave him a burst of energy before dinner.

Your energy window might reveal itself through simple observation: When did I feel surprisingly good today? When did movement feel almost easy instead of like a battle?

The beauty of this approach is that movement doesn't need to be a formal "workout." Taking an extra lap around the supermarket counts. Climbing the stairs slowly while listening to music counts. Stretching while you wait for your coffee to brew counts. The key is tuning into when your body says, "Now feels doable," and using those moments wisely.

Try this: For a few days, jot down quick notes in your phone about when you felt most energetic or when pain was lowest. Note what you were doing and how you felt. You'll likely spot patterns. Maybe mornings work best. Maybe you get a lift after eating. Maybe there's a sweet spot in your schedule you've been overlooking. Once you identify it, protect it. That's your time to move.

Everyday Movements That Count

When I talk about exercise, I'm not talking about CrossFit or marathon training unless that's genuinely your thing. For most of us, especially those dealing with pain or years of being sedentary, the best exercise is simply the one you'll actually do.

Walking remains the gold standard for accessible movement. It's free, it requires no special equipment beyond comfortable shoes, and you can do it almost anywhere. Start with whatever feels manageable, even if that's just to the end of your driveway and back. One of my first "wins" was making it around my block without stopping. A month earlier, I wouldn't have attempted it.

If walking feels tough on your joints, water-based activities can be life-changing. Community pools often have water walking or gentle aquatics classes. The buoyancy takes pressure off your joints while still providing resistance for your muscles. I tried it once during a particularly bad pain flare and was shocked by how good it felt to move freely in the water.

For building strength at home, bodyweight exercises work remarkably well. Wall push-ups, chair squats, and standing leg lifts require no equipment and can be modified to any fitness level. YouTube has countless free videos demonstrating proper form for beginners. Start with just a few repetitions and build gradually.

Some people discover they need the structure of a class. Beginner yoga, chair yoga, or gentle Pilates classes designed for people with limited mobility can provide both guidance and community. Others thrive on informal movement: dancing in the kitchen while making dinner, gardening, playing actively with grandkids, even taking the stairs instead of the elevator.

The Mayo Clinic emphasizes that for people managing weight and metabolic health, the goal is moderate, consistent activity (Mayo Clinic Staff, 2023). That could mean 20-30 minutes most days of the week, but it doesn't have to happen all at once. Three 10-minute walks spread throughout your day count just as much as one 30-minute session.

Why Muscle Mass Is the Quiet Game-Changer

On a GLP-1, muscle is not optional. It's the one thing that decides whether you come out of this journey stronger and metabolically healthier, or smaller but frailer.

When you lose weight on these medications, a meaningful portion of what you lose can be lean tissue, including muscle, not just fat. Recent research suggests that roughly 25% of the total weight lost on GLP-1s comes from lean mass, and in some studies that figure has been even higher, especially in older adults and women (Karakasis et al., 2025; Neeland et al., 2024). Researchers at UC Davis have estimated that 15–25% of weight reduction on these drugs is lean mass, and the proportion is similar to what happens with any rapid calorie restriction. The speed at which GLP-1s work is what makes the issue more urgent than a gradual diet would be (UC Davis Health, 2025).

This matters especially for women in midlife. We already start losing muscle naturally after 40, about 1% per year, and that loss accelerates around perimenopause. Muscle is what keeps metabolism humming, bones loaded and dense, blood sugar stable, and bodies functional with age. Losing too much of it during a year on Wegovy or Mounjaro can mean a lower number on the scale but actually weaker, more insulin resistant, and at higher risk for falls and injury down the road (Endocrine Society, 2025).

The good news is that muscle loss on GLP-1s is not inevitable. It's preventable. The playbook comes down to three things, working together: enough protein, real strength training, and a few smart supplements.

Strength Training: The One Thing That Actually Preserves Muscle

The single most important piece of advice in this chapter: lift weights twice a week. That's the secret to keeping the muscle you have while the fat comes off.

Walking is wonderful for mood, blood sugar, and heart health. But walking will not preserve muscle on a GLP-1. Only resistance does, and the research is unanimous on this point (Karakasis et al., 2025). Without that signal, the body has no reason to hold on to muscle when calories are scarce, and on a GLP-1, calories are always scarcer than the body is used to.

You do not need heavy weights. A pair of 5-pound and 10-pound dumbbells is genuinely all most people need to start. The "you have to lift heavy or it doesn't count" idea is one of the most discouraging myths in fitness, and it stops a lot of women from ever picking up a weight at all. For someone new to resistance training, even light dumbbells will move the needle. Heavier weights can come later, but plenty of women in their 50s and 60s preserve muscle beautifully on 5s, 8s, and 10s.

Twenty minutes, twice a week, with weights you can actually manage. That's the bar. Not an hour at the gym. Not a CrossFit class.

Where to find guidance you can trust

Specific routines are best left to people who do this for a living. A few places worth exploring:

- **Dr. Stacy Sims**, exercise physiologist who specializes in women in midlife and menopause. Her book *Next Level* is the closest thing to a definitive resource for women over 40 on strength training, hormones, and muscle preservation.
- **Caroline Girvan on YouTube**, free follow-along strength workouts that range from absolute beginner to advanced, mostly using dumbbells.
- **Apple Fitness+ or Peloton App**, both have strength programs designed for people starting from zero, with adjustable weights.
- **A trainer for two or three sessions**. Even a few sessions with someone who can show proper form is one of the best investments you can make. Not a long-term commitment, just learning the basics safely.

For chronic pain, find a trainer or program that knows how to adapt around it. Seated dumbbell work, resistance bands while sitting, pool-based strength sessions, and gentle Pilates all count. The form that works for your body is the form that builds muscle in your body.

Protein: The Building Block You Can't Skip

Chapter 8 covered protein in detail: the math, the timing, the food sources. The two chapters connect like this: the protein in Chapter 8 is the raw material; the strength training in this chapter is the signal that tells your body to use it. Without one, the other is wasted.

A few specifics that matter on a GLP-1: research suggests that on these medications, women and older adults tend to lose more muscle if their protein intake is on the low side (Endocrine Society, 2025). Aim for the higher end of the range covered in Chapter 8, 1.2 grams per kilogram of body weight, spread across three to four meals, and prioritize a protein-rich snack or shake within an hour or two of strength sessions. If hitting your number through food isn't realistic because appetite is suppressed (which is half the point of the medication), a daily whey or plant-based protein shake is not cheating. It's the bridge to your target.

Creatine: The Most Underused Tool in Your Toolkit

If protein is the building block and strength training is the signal, creatine is the multiplier. It's the single most evidence-backed supplement on earth that almost no one over 40 is taking, and personally, it's a non-negotiable in my own routine.

Creatine is a compound the body already makes and stores in muscle. Supplementing does three things that matter on a GLP-1: it helps muscles produce energy during strength training so you can train harder, it draws water into muscle cells (creating a more muscle-preserving environment during weight loss), and in studies of older adults and people losing weight, it has consistently been shown to reduce the amount of lean mass lost during a calorie deficit (Candow et al., 2021; Chilibeck et al., 2017).

Here's how simple it is. Take 5 grams of creatine monohydrate daily, with food or in a protein shake. Time of day doesn't matter. No "loading" needed. The cheapest plain monohydrate powder works as well as anything fancier. Brands like Bulk Supplements, Optimum Nutrition, or Thorne all make versions for under $30 that last several months. I take mine mixed into my morning protein shake. It's that easy.

A few common worries: creatine is not a steroid, it doesn't cause bloating in the way you might be thinking (the water it draws goes into muscle cells, not under the skin), and decades of research have shown it's safe for healthy kidneys. Mention it to your doctor before blood work, since it can slightly raise creatinine readings, but that's meaningless if they know you're supplementing. Creatine paired with resistance training also has emerging research showing benefits for bone density, cognition, and recovery, three things that matter more after midlife.

If you do nothing else differently from this chapter, do these three things: strength train twice a week, hit your protein target, and take 5 grams of creatine a day. That combination is the closest thing to a guarantee that the weight you lose is fat, not the muscle you'll need for the next thirty years.

Signs You Might Be Losing Muscle

Even with the best plan, it's worth knowing what muscle loss feels like so you can catch it early. Watch for:

- Strength dropping in everyday tasks. Groceries feel heavier, stairs feel harder, opening jars takes more effort.
- Faster scale loss than expected. Losing more than 2–3 pounds per week consistently after the first month.
- Looking "softer" or "deflated" even as the number drops.
- Persistent fatigue that doesn't lift with rest.

If you notice these, the answer is rarely to quit the medication. It's almost always to slow down the dose escalation, dial up your protein, get more serious about resistance training, and add creatine if you haven't. Talk to your provider about dropping back to a lower dose for a few weeks if needed. The medication still works at lower doses for most people, and a slower, sustainable rate of loss preserves more of what you want to keep.

Movement as Mood Medicine

When you move, your brain releases neurochemicals, such as endorphins, that genuinely lift your mood and help manage stress (Mayo Clinic Staff, 2025). After even a short walk, you might notice you have more patience during family time, or your mind feels clearer for tackling problems.

On my worst pain days, when I couldn't do much physically, I learned that even gentle stretching or a few minutes of deep breathing while doing simple movements could shift my mental state. I wasn't "working out," I was giving my brain and body a chance to reset.

Using activity as a stress break, a happy ritual, or social time tends to be far more motivating than chasing arbitrary numbers on a fitness tracker. When movement connects to feeling good rather than punishing yourself for eating too much or trying to shrink your body, consistency becomes much more natural.

Quick Exercise: Finding Your Energy Window

What it does: This helps you identify the best times for movement based on your actual energy patterns, not what a fitness plan tells you "should" work.

How to do it:

1. For three to five days, track when you have the most energy or experience the least pain. Note your mood and what you're doing in a simple phone note or journal. Don't overthink it, just jot down "felt pretty good around 10 a.m." or "really dragging after lunch."
2. Look for patterns. Do you consistently feel better at certain times? After eating? Before? On days when you've slept well?
3. Choose one gentle or moderate movement that actually appeals to you. Not what you think you should do, but what sounds tolerable or maybe even pleasant. A stroll around your neighborhood, a few minutes of stretching, dancing to one favorite song, light gardening, whatever.
4. Schedule this activity during your identified energy window, even if it's only five to ten minutes. Put it in your calendar like any other appointment.
5. After the activity, take a moment to reflect: How do you feel? Less tired? More motivated? Write down anything positive, even tiny observations like "my back felt looser" or "I felt accomplished."

The goal of this exercise is to gather data about what actually works for your body and your life. Each small win restores confidence and builds curiosity about what movement can bring to your daily experience.

Motivation for the Reluctant Mover

Even when your body feels capable of movement, your mind might throw up a dozen reasons to stay put. I spent years in that space, especially on days when my back pain was screaming. For many of us, especially those who've struggled with weight or fitness for years, exercise carries a lot of emotional baggage.

Maybe you remember feeling judged in a busy gym, or perhaps an old injury left you genuinely worried about getting hurt again. Maybe you've internalized those messages about "no days off" and "no excuses," which creates this impossible standard where you either go all-in or you're a failure. For women, especially, juggling households, careers, and family responsibilities while battling fatigue and self-doubt, these barriers feel even heavier.

Then there's age. Joints feel stiffer than they used to. Old injuries have a way of resurfacing. Your metabolism isn't what it used to be, and comparisons become this constant whisper that tells you improvement is out of reach unless you're already an athlete. The world tells us to push harder, do more, but shame and guilt pile up when unpredictable schedules or a simple lack of motivation get in the way.

I had to completely reframe what exercise meant to break that cycle. It's not punishment for eating. It's not another task to check off some impossible to-do list. It's a gift you give yourself, a daily act of saying, "I'm worth this five minutes. I'm worth this breath of fresh air."

Success stopped being about miles run or pounds lost. Sometimes it was just getting up from my chair to stretch during a long work call. Sometimes it was a silly dance party in my kitchen. The brave choice, I realized, was to value progress over perfection and to celebrate every moment I showed my body that it mattered, no matter how small.

Redefining What Counts

One of my readers, Nora, told me she avoided group fitness classes because she felt self-conscious. But she noticed her mood always lifted during her daily walks with her dog. So instead of forcing herself to join a gym, she made her own ritual: rain boots, a favorite podcast, and quiet time in her neighborhood. That became her exercise, and it stuck because it felt like self-care, not obligation.

Michelle was never a morning person and had given up on traditional workout advice about exercising first thing. She started doing gentle stretches each night while listening to audiobooks. For her, that evening routine became sacred, something she genuinely looked forward to.

Maria found her movement in dancing around her living room after dinner, often inviting her daughter to join. Over time, these spontaneous dance parties became more than exercise; they became joyful memories she was creating with her child while also modeling that moving your body can be fun.

These patterns gave movement meaning and joy instead of dread. That's the key. When you connect physical activity to something positive in your life, whether that's time with your dog, a favorite podcast, bonding with your kids, or just a few minutes of peace, you're far more likely to maintain it.

Starting Small and Stacking Habits

Barriers don't magically disappear, but small actions build confidence in a way that ambitious plans never do. I became a huge believer in micro-goals. Committing to just five minutes of movement, whether that's stretching, walking around the block, or doing a handful of squats while my coffee brewed, was enough to quiet the perfectionist voice in my head that insisted anything less than an hour-long workout wasn't worth doing. Many people find success with "habit stacking," linking movement to everyday anchors you're already doing. Calf raises while brushing your teeth. Shoulder rolls while waiting for the kettle to boil. A few squats during commercial breaks. These tiny additions don't require extra planning or motivation; they just piggyback on existing routines. When low energy or packed schedules threaten your momentum, these small wins remind you that even two minutes count. Every choice stacks up. On my worst pain days, when a walk was out of the question, I'd do some gentle arm circles or stretch my hamstrings while sitting. Not impressive by anyone's standards, but it kept me connected to the habit of moving. It told my brain: we're still doing this, just differently today.

Stories of Breakthrough

Let me share a few more stories that might resonate. Elaine started out genuinely embarrassed at the idea of working out in public. She turned to YouTube workouts at home, where her mistakes and struggles were hers alone. Each session built confidence. Within a few months, she felt ready to try a beginner yoga class at her local community center and was surprised to find herself welcomed, not judged.

Priya used evening walks in her neighborhood to decompress after stressful workdays. Step by step, those walks became meditative, melting away tension and leaving her ready for family time. She wasn't trying to hit a specific step count or burn a target number of calories; she was walking for her mental health, and the physical benefits came along for the ride.

Julie was dealing with significant joint pain when a friend suggested water aerobics. She was skeptical but gave it a try. The gentle resistance and buoyancy made movement feel possible again. After a few months, she built up enough confidence and strength to join a local hiking group, discovering a love for gentle trails and a circle of supportive friends who became an important part of her life.

Using Technology and Community for Support

When your motivation feels shaky, tools can help. Fitness trackers, apps, and online communities help you to tie new habits to reminders and feedback that keep you engaged. Small victories, like earning a badge for a week of activity or getting a reminder to stand up and stretch, can provide the gentle push you need on days when resistance creeps in. Social connection matters too. Sharing your journey with a friend, joining an online challenge, or even just posting your daily walk in a group chat creates accountability without pressure. I found that knowing my neighbor was also walking each morning made it easier to lace up my shoes on days when I really didn't feel like it. We weren't competing; we were just companioning each other in this effort to show up for ourselves.

The main point is this: You don't have to love exercise. You don't have to be naturally athletic. You just have to be willing to find what works for you, start small enough that it feels significant, and trust that consistency, not intensity, is what creates lasting change.

Personalizing Your Fitness Plan With Tech

Once you've started moving more consistently, technology can help you track progress, stay motivated, and fine-tune what's working. But the wearables and fitness apps should serve you, not become another source of stress or obligation. The goal is to use these tools to make progress visible and keep momentum going, not to obsess over hitting arbitrary targets every single day.

Choosing the Right Tools for You

The best fitness tracker is simply the one you'll actually use. If you're curious but hesitant, start simple. A basic pedometer or a straightforward app that quietly counts your steps works fine. No fancy setup, no overwhelming data.

For people who want gentle reminders and the satisfaction of seeing progress, Fitbit stands out. Its interface focuses on simplicity and encouragement, colorful step graphs, friendly nudges to move, and little celebrations when you reach daily goals. The social features let you connect with friends to take on optional challenges if that motivates you.

An Apple Watch integrates fitness more deeply into your daily life, pairing movement tracking with health metrics like heart rate, sleep quality, and even breathing reminders. If you're already in the Apple ecosystem, it feels like a natural extension of your devices.

If you love detailed data and want training-level insights, Garmin provides advanced analytics, including pace, distance, heart rate zones, and performance metrics. It's popular with serious athletes but can be adapted for beginners who are data-curious.

There are also budget-friendly options like Amazfit or simple step-counting phone apps that deliver reliable basics without a learning curve or significant investment. The key is matching your comfort level and budget with a device that feels inviting, not intimidating.

Setting Realistic, Motivating Goals

Once you have your tool, resist the urge to immediately aim for 10,000 steps or any other target the app suggests. Instead, customize goals based on where you're actually starting from. The whole point is to create small successes that build momentum.

Open your app's settings and look for the option to adjust daily targets. Set them low enough to guarantee wins, especially in the beginning. If you're coming from a mostly sedentary lifestyle, maybe you start with 4,000 steps a day. Or track three "stand up and move" breaks during your workday. Or commit to just 10 minutes of intentional activity.

One approach that worked for me: I ignored the preset goals entirely at first and just tracked my baseline for a week. How much was I naturally moving without any particular effort? Once I knew my average, I set my initial goal just slightly higher, maybe 500 more steps per day. That felt doable, and each time I hit it, I got that little dopamine boost of achievement. The trick is letting your tracker be a supportive companion, celebrating every bit of movement without making slip-ups feel like failure. On days when you don't hit your target, that's just information. Maybe you were genuinely busy. Maybe your body needed rest. Adjust and move on.

Using Feedback to Adjust and Improve

The real power of tracking comes from reviewing patterns over time. Most apps have a "Trends" or "History" feature. Check it weekly or monthly to see what your real life looks like, not what your aspirational self wishes it looked like.

You might notice Wednesdays are consistently high-energy days, while Mondays tend to drag. Maybe weekends involve more sitting than you realized. This isn't about judgment; it's about gathering useful data.

Use what you learn to tweak your routines. If weekends are slow, schedule a family walk after dinner. If energy dips every afternoon, set a reminder to move around your house or do a few stretches. If you're plateauing, look for gentle next steps: Add a few flights of stairs once a week, try a slightly longer route on your walk, experiment with a new type of movement.

The Social Side of Fitness Tech

One of the surprises for me was how much fun and motivation came from sharing goals with others. Most trackers have built-in social features: friendly step challenges, virtual high-fives, and circles where you can compare daily activity with friends or family.

Joining or starting a challenge turns healthy routines into something playful rather than pressured. I've heard from people who stuck with walking routines far longer because they joined a month-long step challenge with coworkers. Others found accountability through a private Apple Watch group where friends shared encouragement and gentle ribbing about missed goals.

The social aspect keeps things light. You wake up to emoji-stacked cheers on days when you crushed your goal. You get a friendly nudge when you've been sitting too long. Having people in your corner makes consistency easier and more enjoyable. Just be thoughtful about who you connect with. You want supporters and companions, not competitors who make you feel inadequate. The goal is mutual encouragement, not comparison that breeds stress.

Keeping Technology in Perspective

Over time, the data from your tracker should reduce pressure, not add to it. Ups and downs become part of your story, not evidence that you're failing. Some weeks you'll crush your goals. Other weeks, life will get chaotic, and your step count will drop. Both are okay.

I learned to view my tracker as a tool that celebrates my returns. After a rough week where I barely moved, my device didn't scold me. It just quietly tracked those first few steps when I got back to it, ready to cheer me on again. That non-judgmental support helped me maintain momentum far better than any harsh self-criticism ever did.

Breaking the All-or-Nothing Cycle

Even with the right tools and good intentions, many of us still get stuck when results aren't immediate or routines get disrupted. This is where "all-or-nothing" thinking loves to creep in, and trust me, I know this trap intimately.

For years, my approach to exercise was binary: either I was training hard, pushing through pain, doing everything "right," or I'd given up entirely and wasn't moving at all. There was no middle ground. This mindset got reinforced by fitness culture and decades of diet messaging that insisted success means a flawless journey, that one misstep means starting over or quitting.

The problem with perfectionism is that life doesn't cooperate. Meetings run late. Bodies hurt. Some days, motivation just vanishes. When you're locked in all-or-nothing thinking, these normal hiccups become evidence of failure. You miss two days of walking because of work and exhaustion, and suddenly you've "ruined" everything. The familiar urge is to quit entirely and tell yourself there's no point trying unless every day can be perfect.The Trap of "Dirty" Goals

Researchers studying post-diet culture attitudes discuss "dirty" goals, those built around external approval and the belief that only perfect, outcome-based achievements have real value (Dodier, 2024). These goals make your worth dependent on hitting certain numbers, maintaining perfect streaks, and never stumbling on a rest day or with food choices.

When fitness becomes rigid like this, real life clashes with strict targets, creating pressure that actually blocks resilience. The Mayo Clinic's research on habit formation is clear: lasting change depends on steady, repeated behaviors, even with interruptions, not on single bursts of perfect performance (Noble, 2023). It's the compounding effect of returning to healthy choices, over and over, that protects your progress.

Learning to Spot the Pattern

The first step in breaking the all-or-nothing cycle is learning to catch yourself in the moment. Here's a simple practice that helped me:

When you notice you've missed a workout or "slipped up" somehow:

1. **Pause and describe what happened neutrally:** "I didn't go for my walk today because I had a headache and felt exhausted." No drama, no judgment, just facts.
2. **Notice and name the feeling:** Frustration? Guilt? Disappointment? Just acknowledge it without fighting it.
3. **Reframe it:** "One missed walk doesn't erase the progress I've made. My efforts over the past weeks still count. Tomorrow I'll walk again, or I'll do some stretching today instead."
4. **Choose a tiny next step:** Maybe that's stretching for five minutes right now. Maybe it's taking a short walk around your house. Maybe it's just circling tomorrow's planned activity on your calendar. Something small that reconnects you to the habit without overwhelming pressure.

As you repeat this pattern, new habits grow. You start proving to yourself that returning is what matters, not never falling away in the first place.

Tracking Small Wins

One strategy that worked surprisingly well for me was tracking behaviors rather than outcomes. Instead of obsessing over whether I lost weight that week, I'd track whether I went for my walks, prepped healthy meals, and got decent sleep.

You can do this with an app, a notebook, or even just checkmarks on a calendar. The visual reminder of consistency builds its own momentum.

Small wins compound. Maybe this week you can manage three walks instead of your planned five. That's not failure, that's three more walks than you would've taken if you'd quit. Next week might be four. Or it might be two. The point is you're still showing up, still adjusting, still in the game.

Embracing Flexibility

Real life requires flexibility, especially for those navigating adult responsibilities, hormonal changes, periods of illness, or chronic pain like mine. Some days your body needs rest more than it needs movement. Some weeks, work or family demands every bit of your energy.

Learning to adapt rather than abandon ship is the skill that makes all the difference. Maybe you swap a full workout for a gentle yoga session. Maybe you take a brisk walk instead of a run. Maybe you do five minutes of stretching before bed and call that enough. All of those choices keep you connected to the habit of caring for your body, even when the original plan isn't feasible. Here's a question that helped me shift out of judgment: "What helped me stick to my goal last week, and can I repeat any part of that now?" This moves your focus away from what you failed to do and toward what actually works in your real life.

It's curiosity instead of criticism.

Managing Weight Loss Anxiety and Fear of Regain

Something that doesn't get talked about enough is how, even as you're making progress, anxiety about regaining weight can lurk in the background. If you've been through previous cycles of losing and regaining, that fear makes perfect sense. The emotional toll of weight cycling is real, and "anticipatory anxiety" can undermine your confidence before you've even stumbled.

I worried about this too. What if the medication stops working? What if I regain everything? What if I'm setting myself up for another round of disappointment?

What helped me was treating potential setbacks as data points, not disasters. If my weight plateaus or ticks up a pound or two, that's information. Maybe I need to adjust my eating. Maybe I need more sleep. Maybe my body is just doing what bodies do, fluctuating naturally. It's not evidence that I've failed or that everything is falling apart.

Mental strategies for addressing fear of regain:

- **Visualization:** Spend a few minutes picturing yourself maintaining your health a year from now, five years from now. What does that look like? What habits are you maintaining? Don't focus on a specific number on the scale; focus on feeling capable, strong, and energized. This mental rehearsal helps your brain believe maintenance is possible.
- **Relapse prevention planning:** Set up routine check-ins, whether that's with yourself, a friend, your doctor, or a support group. Decide in advance what you'll do if you notice things slipping. Maybe that's recommitting to tracking your food for a week. Maybe it's scheduling an extra walk with a friend for accountability. Having a "plan B" for stressful situations or travel takes some of the fear out of the equation.

The truth is, fluctuation is normal. Your weight will go up and down a little. Your routines will need adjustment as life changes. People who maintain significant long-term weight loss aren't people who never stumble; they're people who learned to course-correct quickly and without shame.

Building Lasting Motivation Through Non-Scale Wins

As we discussed in Chapter 7, the number on the scale can't be your only measure of success. It's too volatile, too influenced by factors beyond your control, and frankly, it doesn't capture what really matters about this journey. Lasting motivation comes from intrinsic rewards, from noticing and celebrating all the ways your life is improving beyond what a scale can measure. This is the difference between "I want to see a lower number" and "I want to feel healthy and strong." One is external and fragile. The other is internal and resilient.

For me, non-scale victories became the real evidence that change was happening. The first time I bent down to tie my shoe without my back screaming. Or the afternoon I realized I'd been on my feet for hours without thinking about it. Then came the morning I woke up with energy instead of dread. Those moments mattered far more than any number.

Creating Your Non-Scale Victory Tracker

Start noticing and recording these wins. You can use a journal, a note on your phone, or a simple chart. At the end of each week, reflect on what improved:

- Did you sleep better?
- Do you have more energy at certain times of day?
- Are clothes fitting differently or more comfortably?
- Did you climb stairs without getting winded?
- Did you play with your kids or grandkids without your back or knees complaining?
- Did you feel more confident in social situations?
- Did you notice your mood improving?
- Did you accomplish something physically that would've been hard before?

These observations build a powerful case for continuing. When the scale isn't moving but you're sleeping better, moving easier, and feeling stronger, that's real progress. Don't dismiss it.

Rewarding Progress Without Food or Weight Goals

Set up a reward system that celebrates milestones without using food or making it about a number on the scale. Maybe after a month of consistent walking, you buy yourself new walking shoes or that book you've been wanting. Maybe after sticking with your routine through a stressful week, you schedule a massage or take an afternoon completely for yourself.

These rewards reinforce that you're doing something valuable for yourself, not just punishing your body into submission. They help your brain connect healthy behaviors with positive outcomes beyond weight loss.

Revisiting Your "Why"

Motivation evolves. What drives you today might be different from what drove you to start this journey. Check in with yourself regularly: Why does this matter to me right now? What am I hoping to gain or protect?

Some people find it helpful to write themselves a "motivation letter" explaining why they're committed to this path. Others create a vision board or digital collection of images that represent their goals, whether that's hiking with grandkids, traveling comfortably, or simply feeling at home in their bodies.

When motivation dips, which it will, revisit these reminders. They'll help you reconnect with your deeper purpose beyond the day-to-day frustrations.

Cultivating Self-Compassion and Resilience

This might be the most important section in this entire chapter. Everything we've talked about—the movement strategies, the technology, the goal-setting, it all works better when it's built on a foundation of self-compassion rather than self-criticism.

Research consistently shows that self-kindness supports lasting change better than harsh internal criticism (Šoková et al., 2025; Wong et al., 2025). When you beat yourself up for missing a workout or making a food choice you regret, you're not motivating yourself, you're creating stress that actually leads to more setbacks, not fewer.

Daily Self-Compassion Practices

Start each day with a simple reminder: "I'm doing the best I can with what I have today." On tough days, when pain flares or energy is low, tell yourself, "It's okay to need rest. My worth isn't determined by how much I accomplish."

When you catch yourself in harsh self-criticism, pause and reframe: Instead of "I'm so lazy, I skipped my workout," try "I needed rest today. Tomorrow I'll move again."

Some people find mantras helpful: "Progress, not perfection." "Every return is a victory." "I'm building health, not chasing a number."

Building Resilience Through Reflection

At the end of each day, try the "three things that went well" exercise. Write down three things, however small, that went right today. Maybe you chose a healthy lunch. Maybe you took five minutes to stretch. Maybe you just made it through a difficult day without completely derailing your routines. Focusing on what worked, rather than on only what didn't, rewires your brain to notice success rather than only failure.

This practice builds genuine resilience. You start to see setbacks as temporary and specific, not permanent and all-encompassing. A bad day becomes just that, a bad day, not evidence that you're incapable of change.

Look for role models who've overcome adversity, whether that's people in your life or stories you find online or in books. Seeing others navigate challenges and come out stronger reminds you that struggle is part of every successful journey, not proof that you're uniquely flawed.

Knowing When to Seek Support

Sometimes self-compassion and personal strategies aren't enough, and that's completely okay. If you find yourself stuck in patterns of harsh self-criticism, overwhelming anxiety about weight, or behaviors that feel compulsive rather than healthy, consider reaching out for professional support.

Therapy, especially with someone trained in health psychology or eating disorders, can provide tools and perspective that make everything else easier. Coaching can offer accountability and encouragement tailored to your specific situation. Support groups, whether in-person or online, connect you with others who understand the struggle.

There's no shame in asking for help. In fact, recognizing when you need support and actually seeking it out are among the strongest, most self-compassionate things you can do.

Some resources to consider:

- The National Eating Disorders Association (NEDA) offers information and referrals.
- Psychology Today's therapist directory lets you search for professionals specializing in weight, body image, and health behavior change.
- Online communities like Reddit's r/loseit or specialized Facebook groups can provide peer support.
- Many hospitals and health systems offer medical weight management programs with built-in counseling and support.

The journey toward sustainable health isn't meant to be walked alone. Building a team of supporters, whether friends, family, professionals, or peers, makes the path easier and the outcomes better.

Moving Forward With Confidence

Instead of viewing exercise as punishment or your body as a problem to fix, you're learning to see movement as a gift you give yourself and your body as something worthy of care and respect. Instead of demanding perfection, you're embracing consistency and flexibility.

Instead of letting the scale dictate your worth, you're noticing all the ways your life is genuinely improving.

This shift takes time. Some days you'll nail it. On other days, you'll forget everything you've learned and fall back into old patterns. That's normal. That's human. What matters is that you keep returning, keep adjusting, keep showing up for yourself with kindness instead of criticism.

You're building something that lasts, not through force or rigid discipline, but through flexibility, self-awareness, and genuine care for the person you are right now, not just the person you hope to become.

Because real change doesn't announce itself with fireworks. It shows up quietly, in the background, in moments most people will never notice. It's the evening you walk an extra block without thinking about it. It's closing your eyes at night and realizing you're not as exhausted as you used to be. It's choosing to move because it feels good, not because you feel guilty. These are the signs that something inside you is shifting, strengthening, settling into a rhythm you can live with.

If you keep choosing yourself — gently, consistently — strength will come. Energy will come. Confidence will come. Not in a sudden wave, but in small rises that stack and settle until one day you realize you're living in a body that feels more like home than it ever has before.

And as you carry this forward, remember that your progress isn't fragile. It's not something that disappears because of one setback or one tired week. It's built into you now, layer by layer. Every return reinforces it. Every effort, even the smallest one, keeps it alive.

You're not hoping for change anymore. You're creating itpatiently, repeatedly, and that is what lasts.

In the next chapter, we'll move from the big-picture work of staying strong into the small, practical hacks that make this lifestyle stick — the daily routines, tools, and shortcuts that turn willpower into autopilot.

Chapter 10:

Everyday Hacks for GLP-1 Success

Most of us believe that managing a health routine means sacrificing spontaneity, surrendering to rigid schedules, and accepting endless stress. But what if success with GLP-1 medications isn't about strict rules or perfect days? What if it's actually about simple, practical habits woven seamlessly into your daily life, habits that work quietly behind the scenes even on your busiest mornings or during unexpected travel delays?

The real power lies in small hacks and tools that fit the realities of your world, supporting you without overwhelming you. This chapter is about rethinking how everyday choices can build steady momentum, freeing your time and energy so you can focus on living fully, not just managing medication.

"Busy Day" Survival Strategies

The best defense against disruptions in your GLP-1 routine is proactive planning. Life doesn't slow down just because you're working on your health, so you need strategies that work when things get chaotic.

Portable Snacks That Actually Work

Having GLP-1-friendly snacks ready to go means you're never scrambling when hunger strikes and a vending machine is your only option. Think shelf-stable protein sources that can clear airport security: single-serve jerky packs, hard-boiled eggs from home, portable nut butter pouches, and protein powder measured into a shaker bottle.

These fit into work bags without fuss and hold up for hours, giving you steady energy and satiety no matter what your schedule throws at you. For family road trips or evenings shuttling kids around, stash string cheese in an insulated cooler or keep nut mix packs in your car's center console for instant, portion-controlled snacks. When healthy choices are this automatic, you don't have to rely on willpower at your weakest moments.

Airport and Hotel Meal Navigation

Travel used to send me spinning, especially in those early months on Ozempic. But airports and hotels actually offer more options than you'd think for staying on track.

At airport cafes or markets, look for grilled chicken wraps (ditch half the bread for a protein boost), bistro boxes filled with cheese and veggies, and individually packaged hard cheeses. Starbucks cases often have protein boxes, Greek yogurt, and pre-cut veggies, all easy to eat in terminals or on flights.

In hotel breakfast buffets, build your meal with hard-boiled eggs, fresh fruit, and sliced turkey or smoked salmon. If you want something hot, scrambled eggs and plain oatmeal work well, just skip the breakfast breads and pastries. For dinners when you're stuck with only a convenience store or small grocery, grab pre-cooked rotisserie chicken, bags of pre-washed salad greens, or snack-size tuna pouches. Even gas stations usually carry cheese sticks, unsweetened yogurt, and ready-to-eat veggie packs.

The key is focusing on lean protein and produce. This approach keeps your energy steady and your progress intact, even when you're far from your normal routine.

Managing Medication on the Move

Keeping up with injection schedules in new environments calls for reliable reminders. Using your smartphone's alarm or a health app to prompt injections takes the burden off your memory, which can get lost in hectic days.

For crossing time zones on business trips or vacations, adjust your reminder accordingly. If you're shifting more than a couple of hours, consult your healthcare provider about timing your doses safely. I learned this the hard way on a trip to the West Coast, when I wasn't sure whether to inject at my body's usual time or the new local time.

Store your GLP-1 medication in an insulated pouch with ice packs for journeys that stretch into warm weather or involve flights. Keep everything together with needles and alcohol swabs for convenience and privacy. Insulated medical pouches sold online are TSA-compliant and make it straightforward to keep medication cool. Security officers see thermal medical bags all the time. Just declare your medication and ice pack for smooth screening.

At hotels, request a room with a mini-fridge when you book, or ask the staff to store your medication if needed. Most hotels are accommodating about medical needs; you just have to ask.

Discreet Injections in Public Settings

Injecting privately in unpredictable settings doesn't have to be stressful or awkward. On airplanes, I wait for the mid-flight lull when most people are reading or sleeping and head to the lavatory. During late meetings or family dinners, a quick step into a restroom or private office makes injections discreet.

Keep a portable sharps container in your bag for safe disposal. Having all your supplies in a small zipped case means no fumbling around trying to find what you need. The whole process takes less than two minutes once you're comfortable with it.

Movement in Small Time Blocks

Busy days don't have to mean skipped movement. Short, accessible activities between tasks keep your energy up and stress down. Even a few slow desk stretches or ankle circles during long Zoom calls help awaken stiff muscles. A brisk five-minute walk around the parking lot or up a stairwell refreshes both body and mind before your next meeting. Simple routines like ten bodyweight squats or resistance-band pulls can fit in during school pickup or while watching your kid's sports practice.

I've done standing calf raises behind my closed office door more times than I can count. These micro-movements matter for blood sugar stability and overall well-being, even if they don't feel like "real" exercise.

When Things Don't Go According to Plan

Missed meals or injections won't derail your progress if you handle them with composure. When a chaotic workday pushes lunch late or a dose slips by, the first thing to do is check your medication's official guidance for catch-up protocol.

Many practitioners recommend taking the missed injection as soon as you remember, unless it's almost time for your next scheduled dose. Never double up without first checking with your healthcare provider. Most of the time, you just take it when you remember and continue with your regular schedule.

Keep an "emergency kit" with shelf-stable GLP-1-safe snacks, protein shake bottles, string cheese, roasted chickpeas, or nut packs, which lives in your work tote or car glove box. When you miss a meal, you've got backup options that won't spike your blood sugar or leave you feeling terrible.

The most important thing is getting back to your routine at the next meal or dose. Release the guilt and observe what led to the disruption. Use that insight to strengthen your routines going forward. For late nights at the office or school events, prepping portioned, protein-forward meals in advance or batch-cooking on weekends ensures there's always something ready.

Building these everyday strategies into your routine creates a sense of control and reduces anxiety. Knowing a protein snack is stashed in your car or that a mobile reminder will buzz before your dose brings real confidence. These hacks free up mental space and help make your GLP-1 routine an ordinary part of life rather than something that requires constant vigilance.

Integrating GLP-1 Routines With Tech Tools

Busy schedules and shifting priorities make daily consistency feel impossible, even when good intentions are in place. Travel hacks and "survive the chaos" tips only go so far. The next level is building systems that make success the default, no matter how frantic your week gets.

Apps, digital trackers, and smart home gadgets can help your routines run smoothly, whether you're home late, navigating a stack of meetings, or packing for a work trip.

Streamlining Adherence With Smart Apps

Medication adherence starts with simplicity and good reminders. Apps like Medisafe, Apple Health Reminders, and MyTherapy let you set discreet yet reliable alerts for GLP-1 doses and refills, and even for cooling reminders for your injections.

These apps often offer color-coding or tagging options that help distinguish between once-weekly medicine and daily vitamins. Most sync to your calendar, so a missed dose is hard to ignore. For those worried about privacy or sharing devices with family, apps like Medisafe offer settings to lock with a PIN or disable push notifications entirely.

Integrating refill reminders can connect directly to your pharmacy, while export options let you send a data summary or medication log straight to your healthcare team. This streamlines appointments and makes telehealth check-ins more productive.

Food Tracking Made Easier

Food journaling gets less tedious when barcode scanners, photo meal logs, and trend reports make tracking fast and visual. MyFitnessPal offers an enormous food database, so logging a snack or meal is as simple as a scan or a search.

For those more focused on macros or specific nutrients, Carb Manager and Lose It! let you set custom targets, scan packaged food, or search restaurant menus. Photo logging reduces friction, especially when eating out or managing family meals.

These apps usually have export options for sharing food trends with a dietitian, keeping everyone in the loop without endless emails.

I'll be honest, I'm not consistent with food tracking anymore, but in the first few months on Ozempic, it was invaluable for understanding portion sizes and protein intake. Once those patterns became habits, I didn't need to track as closely.

Progress Tracking Beyond the Scale

Smart scales and progress tracking apps round out the digital toolkit. Devices that sync with apps give you precise data on weight, body fat percentage, and other metrics. The companion apps can create daily and weekly reports and sync with Apple Health or other platforms.

This lets you measure the actual impact of your routine changes and simplifies sharing trends during medical appointments. Instead of trying to remember how you've been doing, you can show your provider concrete data that tells the story.

Automating Healthy Decisions

Time-saving technology lifts the pressure to make perfect choices every single day. A programmable rice cooker can batch-prep grains overnight once a week. An air fryer turns leftover chicken into crisp, ready protein in 15 minutes.

Smart home assistants like Alexa can schedule a recurring grocery order. Set up your pantry basics, pre-cut veggies, and favorite snacks to automatically add to your cart each workweek. If you use Google Calendar, set up recurring blocks for meal prep and color-code them to make them stand out.

Even twenty-minute windows to chop veggies or cook chicken breasts save hours of indecision later and make spontaneous takeout less tempting.

Syncing Devices for Better Healthcare

Bluetooth-enabled continuous glucose monitors, smartwatches, and digital kitchen scales can link wellness data so your appointments run more smoothly and adjustments are data-driven.

Devices like Dexcom G7 continuous glucose monitors sync with smartphones and export glucose summaries as email-ready PDFs. Apple Watches and Fitbits track steps, heart rate, and calories burned. Many sync directly with food apps or Apple Health, centralizing everything in one place.

Sending a single file or sharing a summary report means your healthcare team can spot trends, adjust dosages, and support you without long phone calls describing what you think has been happening. The data tells the story more accurately than memory ever could.

If you run into syncing issues, most problems resolve by reinstalling the companion apps, toggling Bluetooth on and off, or updating your device's software.

Managing Tech Overwhelm

Too much information or too many alerts increases stress and actually hurts adherence rather than helping. The key is picking the one or two metrics that matter most during any given season. Tracking steps and weight might work year-round, while monitoring sodium and glucose might take priority after starting a new medication or during a plateau. Mute non-essential notifications in both health and calendar apps. Customize dashboard views to show only your top three trends.

If data starts to feel cluttered, do a digital reset. Archive old logs, streamline your home screens, and revisit which gadgets earn a daily spot on your counter. Not everything needs to be tracked all the time.

The goal of technology should be to reduce mental load, not add to it. If an app or device starts feeling like another chore, step back and simplify.

Real World Shortcuts That Made the Difference

Technology and planning strategies are useful, but some days call for something simpler, something you can feel and taste, something that lands in your real life. The best shortcuts I use blend digital tools with tactile, everyday choices, each designed to lower friction and minimize the need for willpower.

Small Rituals for Big Results

The most pivotal part of my morning, before coffee or checking email, is a glass of water with electrolytes. Nothing wakes me up or resets my mood faster. I grab a tall glass, pour in Berry-flavored LMNT or Nuun tablets, and finish it before taking my medication.

This steady hydration keeps headaches at bay, helps me maintain my fasting window, and prevents the leg cramps that can surface with GLP-1 use. If work pulls me away, a water bottle with a built-in blender ball lets me shake up a dose and sip quietly through back-to-back meetings. As well as keeping me hydrated, this also supplies what my nerves and muscles need before they start complaining.

Many friends have noticed this habit smooths their energy curve through the day, cutting off that 3 p.m. slump and the faint dizziness that signals dehydration. Green powder is my backup for rushed mornings.

Athletic Greens and Bloom have both worked their way into my routine when breakfast choices fall apart. I scoop a serving into cool water, shake, and drink while making lunches for the kids. It doesn't require a blender or fancy ritual, but provides trace minerals my body would otherwise miss.

Even on weekends away or when stress hijacks my appetite, starting my day with a nutrient-rich powder means I don't completely unravel after skipping a meal.

Magnesium glycinate is my fix for restless legs and those spiraling late-night thoughts that sabotage recovery. I keep a small bottle by my toothbrush, take one capsule with water before bed, and let the tension loosen its grip. A few nights each week, when deadlines or family stress keep me awake, I take 1-3 mg of melatonin. The combination isn't every day, just enough to remind my system what real rest feels like.

When I forget these basics, I notice. My mood slips, my patience thins out by afternoon, and my back pain intensifies.

Tools for Physical Comfort

Muscle pain can derail both movement and mindset, so a good heat pack is non-negotiable on tough days. I keep a hospital-grade, weighted heating pad draped over my office chair and use it for 20 minutes after workouts or when I've been sitting at my computer too long.

Standard heating pads never penetrated deeply enough to reach mid-back knots or hip aches. The hospital-grade ones heat up evenly and hold warmth longer, melting tension that might otherwise tempt me to skip my next walk or injection. Having this physical support handy means I don't wait for pain to turn into a full setback.

Travel Hack: Zero Surprises

Traveling often means long lines, late flights, and a parade of sugary temptations. My solution lives in the side pocket of every carry-on: vacuum-sealed beef jerky, mixed nut packets, and a single-serving scoop of whey protein in an old pill bottle.

Once, stranded overnight by a storm, these snacks were the only thing between me and a vending machine dinner of chips and candy bars. On another trip, grabbing a handful of salted cashews in an Uber let me sidestep both a blood sugar crash and airport "deals" on pastries.

These moments are about fast relief that prevents regret and impulsive eating when you're exhausted and hungry.

Anchoring the Routine

While phone alarms and apps make remembering GLP-1 timing easier, life doesn't always run on schedule. I set recurring weekly alarms in my digital calendar for every dose, labeling them with a color unique to my health routines.

There have been times when a work call drowned out the buzz. On those days, I use a physical backup. I keep a sticky note on the fridge or leave the pre-filled injection in my bag close to my keys. The goal isn't just to remember but to prevent the self-blame spiral that sometimes follows a missed dose.

Backups give you room for forgiveness and recovery, not just discipline.

Family Food Made Simple

Sundays in my house mean roasting a batch of chicken thighs, chopping two trays of broccoli, and portioning everything into glass containers. I stash protein in one row, veggies in another, grains and sauces in smaller dishes.

If the week derails with unexpected overtime, sports practice, or a forgotten school assignment, everyone can grab a meal, microwave it, and eat within ten minutes. Shortcut recipes like sheet pan fajitas (chicken, peppers, taco spices) or soy-ginger roasted salmon have saved many evenings from takeout fatigue.

These routines make it possible to eat well when focus is low, energy is drained, and time doesn't cooperate. It's not fancy, but it works.

Rewriting the Inner Script

My biggest mindset hack looks like three words written large in my journal: "Not no, just not yet." This phrase lands hard when I skip a workout, miss a dose by an hour, or say yes to dessert on a day I meant to fast.

Instead of spiraling into defeat, I jot down what pulled me off course: "meeting ran late," "craving comfort after a tough conversation," "just didn't feel like it." Then I end the entry with a plan for the next opportunity: "Walk after dinner tomorrow, set shoes by the door."

This simple practice reroutes guilt into permission, preventing small stumbles from turning into weeks of avoidance. Here's a journaling prompt if you want to try it: "When did you last tell yourself 'not yet'? What will tomorrow's 'yes' look like?"

That question reflects the grace that keeps momentum alive, even when life resists your best intentions.

Making It All Work Together

The beauty of these everyday strategies is that they compound over time. One good choice makes the next one easier. One week of successful meal prep builds confidence for the next. One time bouncing back quickly from a missed dose teaches you that stumbles aren't catastrophic.

You're building a sustainable way of living that supports your health without consuming all your mental energy. That's what makes progress last.

In the next chapter, we'll look at the long view: maintaining your results over months and years, navigating plateaus and setbacks, and building a life where healthy choices are simply what you do, not something you're constantly fighting to maintain.

Chapter 11:

Conquering Obstacles & Plateaus

Nearly half of people on weight-loss journeys experience plateaus where progress stalls despite consistent effort (Owens, 2025). It's one of the most discouraging parts of the process, especially when you're doing everything right.

The scale refuses to budge, or your appetite feels unpredictable, and you start wondering if something's wrong.

Nothing's wrong. This is normal. Understanding why plateaus happen and how to work through them, without losing your mind or your motivation, is what separates short-term results from lasting change.

The Plateau: Why Weight Loss Stalls and What to Do

At first, the pounds shed quickly, and hunger signals seem quieter. Then one day, everything just stops. You're following the same habits, taking your medication as prescribed, eating well, moving your body, and the scale sits there mocking you week after week.

This isn't your imagination, and it's definitely not a sign of failure. It's a real metabolic response driven by your body adapting to carrying less weight.

Why Plateaus Happen

Scientists call this adaptive thermogenesis (Rosenbaum & Leibel, 2010). As you lose weight, your body adjusts to burn fewer calories at rest. Think of it like a smartphone going into low-power mode as its battery drains. Your metabolism shifts to preserve resources, making continued progress less obvious after that initial steep drop.

GLP-1 medications work by reducing hunger and helping you naturally eat less (Health 360, 2025). But as weeks pass, your body learns this new rhythm. Appetite pathways may recalibrate, which researchers describe as a "feedback control system" for body weight. It's like a thermostat, bringing your eating patterns and energy needs toward a new baseline despite the medication.

On top of these internal shifts, old habits can start sneaking back in. Maybe you find yourself reaching for extra almonds when work meetings run late, or pouring a second glass of wine at dinner more often. These are what researchers call "behavioral drift," the natural tendency for old patterns to creep back when stress, travel, or social events nudge routines off course (Sustainability Directory, 2025).

I've experienced this myself. After losing about 15 pounds, my weight stalled for almost a month. I was frustrated and confused because I felt like I was doing everything the same. Looking back, I realized portion sizes had gradually increased, I'd started adding more olive oil to salads without measuring, and I'd gotten less consistent with my evening walks because the weather turned cold.

Identifying a True Plateau

Water weight fluctuates daily due to sodium intake, exercise, and hormones. A true plateau means your weight stays the same for at least three weeks while your daily habits have remained mostly consistent.

Digital scales that show weekly averages, or apps like MyFitnessPal that graph trends over time, offer a clearer view than obsessing over daily ups and downs. Real-world factors that cause temporary stalls include starting a new strength-training routine (muscle soreness causes water retention), traveling across time zones (fluid shifts), or hormonal cycles (bloating and water retention). Check your weight trend over several weeks rather than day by day.

This gives you better insight and keeps anxiety from taking over.

Troubleshooting Checklist to Unstick Progress

When you hit a plateau, approach it like a detective gathering clues, not a judge handing down a sentence. Here's what to check:

1. **Re-evaluate portions and hidden calories:** Are handfuls of nuts getting bigger over time? Have olive oil pours become more generous? Are you drinking calories through lattes, wine, or smoothies? Measure your typical meals and drinks for a few days to get accurate data.
2. **Increase protein or fiber:** Both help with satiety and can modestly boost metabolism. If you're eating 60 grams of protein daily, try bumping it to 80-90 grams. Add more vegetables, beans, or whole grains for fiber.
3. **Modify meal timing:** If you tend to be hungriest in the evening, try moving your largest meal earlier in the day. This doesn't work for everyone, but it's worth experimenting.
4. **Change up your physical activity:** If you've been doing the same workout routine for months, your body has adapted. Try adding resistance training if you've only been doing cardio. If you're already lifting weights, increase the intensity or try a completely different activity. Even bumping your daily step count by 2,000 steps can help.
5. **Check your stress and sleep:** High cortisol from chronic stress and poor sleep both interfere with weight loss. If you're sleeping less than six hours a night or dealing with significant ongoing stress, addressing these issues might be more important than changing your diet or exercise.
6. **Review your medication timing and adherence:** Are you taking your GLP-1 at the same time each week? Missing doses or inconsistent timing can affect results.

The most important thing is patience. Brief stalls are completely normal and don't mean you're doing anything wrong. I've heard from countless people who broke through plateaus after making just one or two small adjustments.

Sometimes the plateau breaks on its own with no changes at all; your body just needed time to recalibrate.

Non-Responder? Troubleshooting Slow or No Results

A small percentage of people see little to no results from GLP-1 medications. This is genuinely rare, but it happens, and it's worth understanding what might be going on.

What "Non-Response" Actually Means

A non-responder is someone who doesn't experience clear appetite suppression or measurable weight loss after several months of consistent, appropriately dosed GLP-1 use. Most people notice appetite changes within days to weeks and see weight trends shift after four to eight weeks.

If you're not seeing any changes after that timeframe, several factors could be at play: genetic differences in how you metabolize the medication, underlying health conditions, such as thyroid problems or high cortisol levels, medication interactions, or simply needing a higher dose or a different GLP-1 formulation.

Systematic Evaluation

Before assuming you're a non-responder, work through this checklist:

1. **Confirm medication adherence and titration:** Are you taking your full prescribed dose consistently? Have you completed the titration schedule your provider recommended, or are you still on a starter dose that might be too low for your body?
2. **Track everything for two weeks:** Keep a detailed log of food, activity, symptoms, stress levels, and sleep. This often reveals hidden patterns. Maybe you're eating more than you realize on weekends. Maybe medication side effects are interfering with nutrition. The data tells the story.
3. **Review liquid calories and hidden intake:** Snacking while cooking, finishing kids' leftovers, sips of juice or soda, extra salad dressing, these "small" calories add up quickly and often go untracked.

4. **Request lab work:** Ask your provider to check thyroid function (TSH, free T3, free T4), cortisol levels, A1C, and liver function. Underlying issues in any of these areas can significantly slow or block weight loss.
5. **Review other medications:** Some medications cause weight gain or interfere with weight loss: certain antidepressants, antipsychotics, steroids, beta-blockers, and insulin can all make losing weight harder.

What to Do If Progress Is Slow

Bring your two-week detailed log to your healthcare provider. Come prepared with specific questions: "Can we adjust my dose?" "Should we try a different GLP-1 medication?" "Are there interactions with my other medications we should address?" Self-advocacy matters here. A simple script: "I've been consistent with my medication and lifestyle changes for X months, but I'm not seeing the appetite suppression or weight loss that's typical. Can we explore next steps together?" Many people have found success after switching from one GLP-1 to another. Ozempic (semaglutide) might not work for you, but Mounjaro (tirzepatide) might. Or vice versa. Each medication has slightly different mechanisms, and individual responses vary.

Avoiding Self-Blame

This is critical: If you're a non-responder or slow responder, it's not because you're not trying hard enough or doing something wrong. It's biology. Your story isn't defined by how quickly the scale moves or whether the first medication you try is the right fit.

I've heard from people who struggled on one GLP-1 for months, switched to another, and suddenly everything clicked. Others found success by combining medication with therapy to address emotional eating patterns they didn't realize were sabotaging their efforts. Some discovered underlying health issues that, once treated, allowed weight loss to finally happen.

Non-response is rare, and even if your first approach isn't working, there are options. The journey isn't over; it might just look different from what you expected.

Coping With Negative Self-Talk and Weight Stigma

When progress slows or stalls, the voice in your head often gets loud and mean.

I'm failing again.

Maybe I'm just meant to be this way.

Why can't I do what others seem to handle easily?

These thoughts aren't random. They echo old wounds: comments from family at holidays, offhand jokes from friends, cold language from healthcare providers, decades of diet culture messaging that your worth is tied to your weight.

Identifying Internalized Weight Bias

Internalized weight stigma doesn't come out of nowhere. Media and health campaigns push the narrative that weight is purely a matter of personal choice and willpower. When you've internalized that message, every setback feels like proof you're weak or lazy or lacking in character.

Research shows that even mental health professionals often hold bias against people in larger bodies, viewing them more negatively and sometimes treating their struggles as character flaws rather than complex health issues (Philip et al., 2025). When you're already fighting your own critical inner voice, encountering this bias in the world makes everything harder.

Cognitive Restructuring

When you catch yourself in harsh self-talk, pause and challenge it. Ask yourself: "What would I say to a close friend in this exact situation?" You'd likely offer kind, rational encouragement instead of blunt judgment. Write down what you'd tell your friend, then read it back to yourself. This simple practice helps weaken the narrative that equates your worth with your weight or the speed of your results.

Here are some self-compassion scripts to try when judgment takes over:

- "I'm allowed to be frustrated, but I'm also allowed to be patient. This process is about health, not punishment."
- "Setbacks are part of every journey. My effort today counts, even if the scale stands still."
- "My body is responding in its own time. I'm learning what works for me, not comparing myself to others."

Journaling for Mindset Shifts

Try this prompt: "When things feel slow, what would I want a wise friend to remind me? How can I keep the bigger picture in view?"

Write freely without editing yourself. These small practices build resilience that helps you return to your goals after setbacks rather than abandoning ship entirely.

Handling External Stigma

Medication-based weight loss sometimes gets dismissed as "taking the easy way out" or "cheating." Well-intentioned but insensitive comments from coworkers, relatives, or even healthcare professionals can quickly undermine your motivation.

Here are some response scripts for navigating intrusive questions or shaming remarks:

- "GLP-1s are part of my medical treatment plan, just like anyone managing a chronic condition. I'm following my doctor's guidance."
- "Weight management is personal. I'd appreciate your support as I work with my healthcare team."
- "I prefer to keep those details private, but thank you for your concern."

Practice these responses, even alone, so you're prepared when comments catch you off guard. You don't owe anyone an explanation for your healthcare decisions.

Finding Supportive Communities

Tackling this journey alone makes setbacks and stigma feel heavier. Connecting with supportive communities significantly lightens the emotional load.

Look for online spaces rooted in body positivity and science-driven approaches. Forums, dedicated social media groups, or hashtags like #GLP1Journey or #HealthAtEverySize can help. Seek out communities with clear ground rules about empathy and respect.

Quality in-person groups may be available through hospital networks, pharmacies, or local health initiatives. When joining any group, notice whether conversations leave you feeling encouraged and less alone, or whether they increase anxiety and comparison.

One community member shared: "After years of hiding my struggles, saying them out loud in a support group showed me I'm not weak or lazy. Others get it, and that's changed how I show up for myself."

Peer validation creates space for healing and makes resilience contagious.

Celebrating Non-Scale Victories to Stay Motivated

We covered non-scale victories back in Chapter 7 and touched on them again in Chapter 9, so I won't repeat everything here. But it's worth emphasizing their importance when you're stuck in a plateau or dealing with slow progress.

When the scale won't budge, NSVs prove that your health is still moving in the right direction. Better sleep, reduced medication, more energy, improved mood, lower blood pressure, clothes fitting better, and less joint pain; these victories are just as important as the number on the scale, sometimes more so.

Using NSVs During Plateaus

Plateaus happen to everyone. NSVs work like fuel to keep you going when the scale gets stubborn. If your weight hasn't changed in three weeks, look back at other markers of progress.

Did your cholesterol numbers improve? Can you carry heavy groceries without getting winded? Did you sleep through the night for the first time in months?

That's proof things are changing under the surface, even if the scale hasn't caught up yet.

I've heard from people who spent weeks stalled on the scale but noticed they needed less blood pressure medication, their rings fit again, they had fewer migraines, or they powered through a busy workday without the usual afternoon crash. They celebrated those "invisible" wins, stayed consistent, and eventually the scale started moving again, too.

Setting NSV-Based Goals

Instead of only focusing on weight loss goals, set goals based on how you want your life to improve:

- Walk a 5K with your family.
- Get seven hours of sleep four nights a week.
- Reduce your A1C by one point.
- Play actively with your grandkids without needing a break.
- Go hiking on a trip you've been planning.

These goals connect to life outside the bathroom scale and give you concrete reasons to keep going, even when progress feels invisible.

For more on tracking and celebrating NSVs, revisit Chapter 7, where we covered this in detail.

Moving Forward With Obstacles

Plateaus, non-response, negative self-talk, external stigma—these obstacles are real and challenging. But they're also navigable. Understanding that plateaus are a normal part of your body's adaptation helps reduce frustration and self-judgment.

You're not on this journey to achieve perfection. You're building sustainable habits that support your long-term health and well-being. Some weeks will show dramatic progress. Other weeks will feel like treading water. Both are part of the same journey.

What matters most is that you keep showing up, keep adjusting, keep treating yourself with the same compassion you'd offer someone you love. The scale will eventually catch up with your efforts. In the meantime, trust the process and notice all the other ways your life is improving.

In the next chapter, we'll dive into the long-term picture: maintaining your results over time, building sustainable habits that last, and creating a life where healthy choices are simply what you do, not something you're constantly fighting to maintain.

Chapter 12:

Side Effects Survival Guide

The first week on a new medication was tougher than I expected. Mornings arrived with a queasy stomach, making even the thought of breakfast unappealing. By mid-morning, my head throbbed just enough to distract me from work, and an overwhelming tiredness settled like a fog that coffee couldn't lift. I was juggling meetings, errands, and family demands, all while feeling off balance.

The side effects were my body's way of telling me something was changing. For many people in midlife, these early hurdles feel more challenging than anticipated, with symptoms that linger just long enough to make daily life feel heavier than usual. Understanding what's happening and knowing when to push through versus when to ask for help makes all the difference.

Evidence-Based Relief for Nausea, Headaches, and Fatigue

Starting a GLP-1 medication when you have a packed schedule, meetings to run, meals to prep, school drop-offs, and workouts planned, can feel overwhelming when side effects hit. Understanding the timeline and having practical strategies ready helps you navigate these early weeks without derailing your entire life.

What to Expect and When

Nausea often appears first, peaking during the initial three to seven days of a new or increased dose. Some people describe it as low-level queasiness that flares after the first morning bite. Others feel waves during the afternoon. Severity typically lessens after the first two weeks as your body adapts. By week three, most people notice real improvement, though lingering mild nausea can persist, especially if you increase your dose or stress interferes with your routines.

You're more likely to experience intense nausea if you have a history of motion sickness, migraines, or tend to skip meals regularly (Zambon, 2020).

Headaches frequently accompany nausea, often showing up in those same first few days and weeks. These aren't typically drilling, light-sensitive migraines, but more tension-based, tightness across the forehead or the back of your neck. Hydration levels, sleep quality, caffeine withdrawal, and hormonal shifts (hello, perimenopause) can make these headaches worse, particularly for women between 40 and 65.

Dose increases, missed meals, or disrupted sleep can bring headaches back after they start to fade (Zambon, 2020; Villaines, 2025).

Fatigue rounds out this trio. It feels like dragging yourself through wet sand, energy dips that creep in by mid-morning or late afternoon. This tiredness can last anywhere from days to a few weeks. If you're in perimenopause or dealing with anemia, thyroid issues, or chronic fatigue syndrome, GLP-1s might amplify your baseline tiredness (Villaines, 2025).

Who Gets Hit Hardest

Symptom severity doesn't affect everyone equally. Women, particularly in midlife, tend to notice side effects more intensely. Age, hormonal fluctuations, existing headaches or migraines, and baseline hydration all make a difference.

Larger starting doses or faster dose increases can make side effects sharper, while those who naturally eat irregular meals or skip breakfast are more vulnerable to stomach upset (Zambon, 2020).

Home Relief That Actually Works

For headaches and fatigue, hydration is critical. Aim for 8 to 10 cups (about 2 to 2.5 liters) of water daily, sipping steadily throughout the day rather than gulping all at once. Add an electrolyte drink in the afternoon, look for low-sugar options like LMNT, Nuun, or unflavored Pedialyte packets. These help your body retain fluids and maintain the balance of sodium, potassium, and magnesium, which often gets disrupted in the early days.

Keep a water bottle on hand and set phone reminders if needed. This simple habit made a massive difference for me, cutting my headaches by at least half.

For nausea, meal timing is your best friend. Before getting out of bed, nibble a few nuts or a protein bite. Keeping your blood sugar steady by eating small, protein-rich snacks every three hours prevents long stretches with an empty stomach, which can worsen queasiness. Stick to gentle foods: yogurt, hard-boiled eggs, salty crackers, or apple slices. Space your main meals out and avoid high-fat or overly sweet foods in the morning (Zambon, 2020).

Build a portable nausea kit. Toss a few ginger chews, acupressure sea bands, and unscented wet wipes into your bag. Keep disposable bags handy during commutes. Some people swear by frozen grapes or lemon slices for easy, refreshing bites on the go.

For headaches specifically, cold packs across your forehead or neck help. Try a five-minute breathing exercise (plenty of free apps available) or gentle stretches like neck rolls and shoulder shrugs. Head outside for a brisk ten-minute walk or take a break from screens. These small interventions can ease tension-type headaches without medication.

For fatigue, gentle movement paradoxically helps more than rest sometimes. A short walk, some light stretching, or even just standing up and moving around your house for five minutes can shift your energy. Don't push hard workouts when you're exhausted, but don't assume complete rest is always the answer either.

Over-the-Counter Medications

Acetaminophen (Tylenol), up to 650 mg every four to six hours, is usually safe for headaches or low-grade pain. Always check with your healthcare provider first and avoid exceeding 3,000 mg per day.

Skip NSAIDs like ibuprofen or naproxen if you have any stomach pain or GI symptoms. These can increase the risk of irritation or ulcers when combined with GLP-1 side effects (Villains, 2025).

When to Request Prescription Help

Reach for prescription anti-nausea medication if vomiting prevents you from staying hydrated or you're unable to keep fluids down twice in 24 hours.

This is essential for preventing dehydration, especially if fatigue worsens or dizziness occurs (Zambon, 2020). A quick call to your doctor or a telehealth provider can get you the support you need. Don't try to tough it out. Getting ahead of severe nausea is far easier than recovering from dehydration.

Gut Health Management on GLP-1s: Preventing Constipation and Digestive Discomfort

After early side effects start improving, you might find your digestive system still feels sluggish. Headaches fade, nausea eases around meals, yet days pass with uncomfortable bloating and constipation. This surprises many people, but it's a predictable experience with GLP-1 medications.

Why It Happens

GLP-1 receptor agonists slow down the movement of food from your stomach to your small intestine, a process called delayed gastric emptying. Food, fluids, and everything that follows move more slowly, which means the urge to have a bowel movement gets delayed and fullness lingers much longer. This is a dose-related effect, well-documented and expected in everyone taking these medications (Chesak, 2025). It's not something you're doing wrong.

Gut side effects tend to show up within the first one to three weeks of starting or increasing your dose. Women in midlife may notice this more because the gut tends to get sluggish as estrogen levels change, compounding the medication's effect.

Prevention and Management Plan

Hit your fiber and water targets. Aim for 25 to 30 grams of fiber daily, focusing on a mix of soluble and insoluble sources. Load up on raspberries, blackberries, chia pudding, overnight oats, and leafy greens. Ready-to-go options like Thorne fiber powder in a shake or Fiber One gummies work for busy days.

Fiber needs water to work properly. Set a personal target of at least 64 ounces (two liters), but two to three liters is ideal (Chesak, 2025). Break it up: a cup first thing in the morning, another at each meal, and one before bed. Set phone reminders if that helps.

Move your body regularly. Even a brisk 10-minute walk after dinner, a few laps around the block midday, or gentle yoga (cat-cow stretches or spinal twists) gets your digestive tract moving. On days packed with meetings, set calendar alerts as cues to stretch or walk. Some people find that linking a fiber-rich snack to mid-afternoon, right before the typical energy slump, helps establish a consistent routine.

Safe Supplements and OTC Options

When the basics aren't enough, over-the-counter options can help (Xing & Soffer, 2001):

- **Magnesium oxide** (400 mg at bedtime) is gentle, unless you have kidney problems. Magnesium citrate is another option that works similarly.
- **Polyethylene glycol** (like MiraLAX) draws water into the colon without causing dependency, so it's safe for short-term use.
- **Stool softeners** like docusate sodium may help when things feel dry, but use them occasionally and check with your provider first.
- **Probiotics** get lots of attention. Look for formulas containing Bifidobacterium lactis. Start with a low dose and track your response for two weeks to find what works best for you.
- **Avoid stimulant laxatives** like senna or bisacodyl for regular use. They can lead to dependency and rebound symptoms over time. Steer clear of high-sugar "detox" gummies, too.

Less Common Symptoms

Bloating, gas, and reflux happen to some people. If these bother you, try skipping carbonated drinks, beans, and heavily processed snacks. Sit up straight while eating, chew slowly, and avoid lying down right after meals. Propping the head of your bed up by a few inches can help minimize reflux overnight.

Small shifts, timing your water intake, choosing fiber-rich snacks, and squeezing in short walks add up to steady gut comfort and better energy throughout your day.

Appetite, Taste Changes, and Food Aversions: Adapting Your Diet

Appetite and taste changes often go hand in hand with the slowed digestion many people experience on GLP-1s. These medications alter how your gut communicates with your brain about hunger and fullness. Messages that normally tell you when you're hungry, what sounds tasty, or how much you want to eat become less clear, leaving you with mixed or muted cravings. This isn't in your head. Research connects these effects to changes in gut-brain signaling (Avcilar, 2022).

What Changes Look Like

For many, appetite shifts run from a simple loss of interest in meals to strong aversions to foods you once loved. You might crave lighter, plainer options like toast, plain rice, or crackers while feeling inexplicably turned off by things you used to enjoy.

The smell of bacon might make you feel queasy. Creamy pasta dishes feel too heavy. Cookies taste overwhelmingly sweet. Fries seem almost greasily enough to coat your mouth. Your usual morning coffee could seem too strong or bitter.

Certain textures or strong flavors, such as garlic, onions, or very spicy food, might spark instant nausea. Meals heavy on cheese, butter, cream sauces, or anything fried are typically "off-limits" because these foods are slower to leave the stomach and can easily trigger fullness or aversion (Avcilar, 2022).

Adapting What's On Your Plate

Stick to bland, soft, or simple foods during tough stretches. Rotate meal elements to avoid monotony. Instead of plain toast every morning, try a poached egg on top or add a bit of smoked salmon for protein and variety. Chicken-and-rice or steamed veggies with a squeeze of lemon become reliable standbys.

Experiment with flavor tweaks. Add fresh herbs, use a splash of vinegar or a squeeze of lemon for brightness, or toss soft foods with a touch of olive oil and chopped green onions for texture. Crunch can help too: cucumber rounds, lightly toasted sourdough, or thinly shaved carrots liven up gentle meals.

Safe Foods and Gentle Meal Ideas

Here are options that many people tolerate well:

- plain rice with steamed veggies
- poached, scrambled, or soft-boiled eggs
- Greek yogurt (unsweetened or lightly sweetened)
- applesauce or baked apples
- frozen grapes, watermelon cubes, or cantaloupe
- cottage cheese with sliced peaches or berries
- avocado smashed on toast
- steamed potatoes with a sprinkle of sea salt
- chicken or veggie broth with tiny noodles or rice
- lightly cooked oatmeal with a drizzle of honey or a sprinkle of cinnamon

Cooling foods like chilled melon, cucumber slices, or popsicles often feel soothing, especially during bouts of nausea or taste fatigue. Keep options simple and hydrating (Avcilar, 2022).

"Reset" Meals for Difficult Days

On rough days, have go-to meals that are easy to digest and comforting: soft scrambled eggs with toast, chicken or vegetable broth with a handful of small pasta, or a plain baked potato with a bit of yogurt. These provide calories, protein, and enough blandness to feel safe when everything else seems overwhelming.

Maintaining Balanced Nutrition

Getting enough nutrients can get tricky with food aversions. Protein shakes, bought or homemade, bridge the gap. Stir in a scoop of collagen or use protein-enriched oat milk in smoothies with soft fruits and spinach. Swap regular yogurt for high-protein options, and consider adding nut butters or flax oil to smoothies for extra calories and nutrients when appetite is low.

Keep an eye on fiber and micronutrients: bite-sized cherry tomatoes, bell pepper strips, or individual nut butter packs are easy additions.

If you notice weight dropping, dehydration symptoms, or energy levels tanking for more than a week, reach out to your healthcare provider or a registered dietitian. Gentle, steady nutrition matters more than perfection, and getting support early prevents bigger problems down the line.

Red Flags: When Side Effects Mean It's Time to Call Your Provider

Most side effects are uncomfortable but not dangerous. They improve with time and basic management strategies. However, some symptoms require immediate medical attention. Knowing the difference can prevent serious complications.

Urgent Symptoms Requiring Immediate Care

Call your provider right away or seek emergency care if you experience:

- **Persistent vomiting or inability to keep fluids down:** If you can't keep down water or other fluids for more than 12-24 hours, you risk dehydration. Signs of dehydration include extreme thirst, dark urine, dizziness when standing, rapid heartbeat, and confusion.
- **Severe abdominal pain, especially with fever:** While some stomach discomfort is normal, severe pain (especially in the upper right abdomen), particularly when accompanied by fever, nausea, and vomiting, could indicate gallbladder problems or pancreatitis, both of which require immediate evaluation.

- **Rapid heart rate or persistent dizziness:** Occasional mild dizziness when standing up quickly can be normal, especially if you're dehydrated. But a heart rate consistently above 100 beats per minute at rest, or dizziness that doesn't improve with hydration and rest, needs medical attention.
- **Vision changes:** Blurred vision or difficulty seeing that doesn't improve could indicate blood sugar issues or other serious problems.
- **Severe allergic reactions:** Difficulty breathing, swelling of the face or throat, or widespread hives require immediate emergency care.

Expected Side Effects vs. Serious Problems

- **Expected and self-limiting:** Mild to moderate nausea for one to three weeks, tension headaches for the first week or two, temporary fatigue, constipation that responds to fiber and water, mild bloating or gas, temporary taste changes or food aversions.
- **Concerning and requiring provider contact:** Vomiting that prevents hydration, weight loss of more than two to three pounds per week consistently, inability to eat for more than two to three days, severe persistent headaches that don't respond to usual treatments, signs of dehydration, worsening fatigue that interferes with daily function, and severe constipation lasting more than a week despite interventions.
- **Documenting Symptoms for Provider Conversations**

Keep a simple symptom diary if you're having ongoing issues. Note:

- date and time symptoms occur
- severity on a scale of 1-10
- what you ate or drank before symptoms
- what helps or makes it worse
- how long symptoms last
- any other relevant factors (stress, sleep, activity level)

This information helps your provider determine whether what you're experiencing is expected or needs intervention.

Scripts for Communicating With Your Healthcare Team

When calling or messaging your provider, include:

"I started [medication name] on [date] and am currently taking [dose]. I'm experiencing [specific symptom] that [describe how it affects daily life]. I've tried [list what you've already done to manage it]. The symptom is [getting better/staying the same/getting worse]. I'm calling because [state your concern or question]."

Example: "I started Ozempic three weeks ago and am taking 0.5 mg weekly. I'm experiencing constant nausea that makes it hard to eat or work. I've tried eating small, frequent meals, drinking ginger tea, and using sea bands, but nothing is helping.

The nausea hasn't improved at all. I'm calling because I can barely keep food down, and I'm worried about getting dehydrated."

Trust Your Instincts

If something feels wrong, call. You're not being dramatic or wasting anyone's time. Healthcare providers would much rather hear from you early when problems are small and fixable than deal with emergencies that could have been prevented.

Better safe than sorry isn't just a cliché. It's genuinely the right approach when starting any new medication. Your instincts about your own body are valuable data. If you feel like something is off, that's worth investigating.

Your Side Effects Toolkit

Side effects are temporary for most people. The nausea fades, headaches improve, your gut adjusts, and taste changes often normalize within a few weeks to months. Some people sail through with minimal issues. Others have a rougher time but find relief with the strategies outlined in this chapter.

The key is having realistic expectations, knowing what tools to use when, and understanding when to ask for help. You're not supposed to suffer through severe symptoms. You're not supposed to tough it out when something feels seriously wrong.

Pay attention to your body, use the strategies that work for you, and don't hesitate to reach out to your healthcare team when you need support. That's not weakness, it's smart healthcare management.

In the next chapter, we'll look at the long view: maintaining your results over time, adjusting your approach as life changes, and building a sustainable way of living that supports your health for years to come.

Chapter 13:

The Road Ahead: Long-Term Success and the Future of GLP-1s

"I don't know why the weight always finds its way back," a friend confessed, frowning at jeans that once fit perfectly but now felt snug. "I did everything right, tracking meals, staying active, taking my medication. But after a while, it's like my body forgets and old habits sneak in without me noticing."

She wasn't alone. Many people using GLP-1 medications for weight loss feel a similar mix of hope and challenge as they move beyond initial results. The journey doesn't end when the pounds drop. In some ways, that's just the beginning. New questions emerge: How do you maintain steady progress without constant struggle? What happens when hunger returns or life disrupts your routine? What does long-term success actually look like?

This chapter explores those realities, offering practical guidance for maintaining what you've worked hard for and navigating the path ahead.

Maintaining Weight Loss: Life After the "Appetite Reset"

After the initial appetite reset with GLP-1 medications, old routines and familiar food thoughts begin to reappear. Hunger may nudge back. Social events present temptations. Former patterns try to resurface. Maintenance is never autopilot; it's responsive, flexible, and constantly evolving.

Smart Weight Trend Monitoring

Long-term success rarely comes from daily weigh-in anxiety or chasing a single perfect number. Think of monitoring as reading trends, not triggers.

A Bluetooth-enabled scale that syncs with Apple Health or MyFitnessPal reveals weekly or monthly weight trajectories. This lets you notice a gentle uptick before it becomes stressful. For some, comfort isn't in data but in a favorite pair of jeans, a ring that fits, or energy levels on walks. Combining subjective self-checks with objective trends provides a safety net without perfectionism.

Early intervention matters most when habits drift for more than seven to ten days or you notice weight trending up two to four pounds. Action steps can be simple: use app reminders to plan a grocery order, schedule a meal prep session on the weekend, or message an online support group for accountability.

These small interventions interrupt "well, I'm off track now" thinking and get you back to center without drama. Consider journaling mood-food connections or changes in hunger in a wellness app if hunger returns faster than expected (García-Gorrita et al., 2025).

Advanced Meal Planning for the New Normal

The maintenance phase requires more than just strict calorie counting. It's about learning how to expand food variety, honor cravings in small doses, and socialize without losing progress. To reintroduce foods you've been avoiding, try this three-step approach:

1. **Add one new item at the start of the week.** Use a food scale or tracking app to determine a portion size aligned with maintenance, not loss.
2. **Eat the new food slowly, checking in with fullness after each bite.** Pause halfway to ask yourself: "Is this as satisfying as I hoped?"
3. **Track your weight, mood, and hunger over the next 48 hours.** If everything stays stable, this becomes a regular option. If not, adjust the portion or timing.

When dining out, review menus in advance and choose grilled, roasted, or steamed proteins first. Then add a starch or dessert if you're truly hungry, not just because others are. Ask for sauces on the side or plan to take half home before you start eating.

If dinner turns into a social event and you eat more than planned, avoid guilt spirals. Plan a lighter lunch or an extra walk the next day rather than cutting meals or overcorrecting.

This protects the trust you're building with your body.

Handling Emotional Obstacles

Many people fear regaining weight more than they feared being heavy in the first place. The drift back to restriction, skipping meals, avoiding favorite foods, or all-or-nothing thinking, often signals anxiety, not actual failure.

Practice "pause strategies" when cravings strike: set a timer for ten minutes, step outside for air, or write down three things you're grateful for about your progress. These mindful techniques create distance from impulsive eating.

If a rough patch lasts, review your data. Look at hunger, mood, and scale numbers for the past month. Search for patterns rather than assigning blame.

Sometimes all it takes is resetting bedtime routines, checking supplement levels, or reaching out for accountability to quiet persistent "I blew it" thoughts.

Tapering Off GLP-1s: Safe Strategies and Relapse Prevention

As concerns about cost, side effects, or desire for less reliance on medication arise, considering a taper makes sense. But this decision needs careful planning and medical guidance.

When and How to Discuss Tapering

Bring these questions to your provider:

- Are my habits stable for at least six months?
- Is my eating manageable with minor hunger fluctuations?
- What's the plan if weight returns?

It's important to agree on shared goals and a slow, stepwise reduction.

A safe protocol means reducing your dose by the smallest possible increments every three to four weeks. During this time, watch for new hunger, mood dips, or energy dips. Logging these changes in your wellness app boosts awareness and helps you catch problems early.

Prepare "emergency" foods like prepped grilled chicken, chopped raw vegetables, or yogurt cups to avoid quick, less mindful choices when hunger increases.

Building Relapse Prevention Systems

Relapse isn't failure, but forgetting to use backup systems makes recovery harder. Keep meal plans for busy weeks saved in your phone and set up a friend for text check-ins. You should always have two or three healthy "grab and go" foods available.

Spotting self-sabotage early, ignoring trends, and drifting from routines mean you can course-correct gently rather than by panicking.

Coping With the Emotional Side of Tapering

Tapering can bring up fears about losing control or regaining weight. These feelings are normal. Some people find it helpful to work with a therapist during this transition, especially if past weight cycling has created anxiety.

Remember that needing to restart medication isn't failure. GLP-1s can be used intermittently or long-term, depending on individual needs. Some people taper successfully and maintain independently. Others find they do better with ongoing medication support. Both paths are valid.

The Next Generation: Emerging Treatments and What's Ahead

The field of metabolic medicine is evolving rapidly. Understanding what's coming helps you make informed decisions about your long-term treatment.

New Medications in Development

Dual and triple agonists are delivering strong results. These medications target multiple hormone pathways at once. Tirzepatide (Zepbound) is now widely used as a GLP-1/GIP dual agonist, and newer triple agonists that also activate the glucagon receptor are showing even greater weight loss in recent clinical trials.

Oral GLP-1 medications are already available, with pills like oral semaglutide offering a needle-free option. Newer, higher-dose oral formulations designed specifically for weight loss are now in late-stage trials and may match the effectiveness of injections.

Longer-acting versions with fewer injections are underway. Researchers are testing once-monthly and bi-weekly GLP-1 formulations that provide the same appetite control with far more convenience for long-term use.Personalized Medicine Approaches

Future treatment will likely involve predicting individual response based on genetic markers, gut microbiome analysis, and metabolic profiles. This could help providers identify which medication and dose will work best for each person before starting treatment, reducing the trial-and-error period.

Digital health tools will increasingly integrate with medical care. Continuous glucose monitors paired with AI algorithms could provide real-time feedback on food choices. Smart scales and activity trackers will share data directly with healthcare teams for more responsive care.

Changes in Guidelines and Access

As evidence accumulates and medications become more established, insurance coverage is expected to improve.

Guidelines from major medical organizations continue to evolve, recommending earlier intervention with GLP-1s for weight management.

Public acceptance is also shifting. As more people use these medications successfully and celebrities openly discuss their use, stigma around medication-assisted weight loss is decreasing.

Combination Therapies

Research is exploring combinations of GLP-1s with other medications: muscle-preserving drugs to maintain lean mass during weight loss, medications that target specific aspects of metabolism, and therapies that address the underlying causes of obesity, such as chronic inflammation (*New GLP-1 Therapies*, 2025). The future is likely to involve personalized combinations tailored to individual needs rather than one-size-fits-all approaches.

Building Your Personalized GLP-1 Blueprint for Lifelong Health

No two GLP-1 journeys look the same. What sets you up for long-term success is keeping your blueprint flexible, not fixed. Your plan should adjust as you do, when your work schedule shifts, you travel more, menopause affects your body, or your health goals evolve.

Regular Self-Audits

Once a month, review your routine with practical questions:

- Are my go-to snacks still working for my hunger and schedule?
- Has my fitness tracker or app outlived its usefulness, or am I ready to try new features?
- Am I meeting my movement goals, or do I need to adjust timing or type of exercise?
- Are my meal choices right for my current energy needs?
- Do my hydration and protein goals align with how my body feels now?

- Is my support team diverse enough to cover questions, encouragement, and accountability?
- Has work, family, or health changed enough that my plan needs to be refreshed?
- Am I tracking mood, sleep, and energy to spot new patterns?

Journals, food diary apps, and smart wearables make tracking streamlined and low-pressure. Even busy weeks offer moments while waiting for coffee or after school drop-off to glance at progress.

Assembling Your Support Team

Think of support as three essential circles:

- **Medical:** Your primary care provider, GLP-1 prescriber, telehealth options, and a registered dietitian all play unique roles. After major life changes, you might need your prescriber to reassess side effects or adjust prescriptions. A dietitian can help when cravings change or meal times shift.
- **Social:** Wellness-minded friends, family members who respect your goals, and fitness buddies turn solo commitment into shared celebration. Walking groups, workout partners, or simply friends who understand your journey provide crucial support.
- **Digital:** Online GLP-1 communities, data-driven health apps, and workout streaming services fill gaps between appointments. These resources offer recipe swaps, a space to vent about setbacks, and motivation during tough times.

After big life events—moving, kids leaving home, menopause symptoms, shifting eating habits—don't hesitate to update this team. You might switch gyms for a better location or restart coaching sessions with a different specialist who offers more targeted advice.

Staying Agile Through Setbacks

Major disruptions, from injuries to medication changes to unexpected life stress, require adaptation. A runner who shifted to low-impact strength training after an ankle injury discovered new favorite workouts.

Someone facing medication side effects adopted an elimination diet approach with their dietitian, tracking potential food triggers one by one until finding relief. Asking for help and trying new approaches isn't backsliding but building mastery.

The Power of Personalization

Research shows that personalized nutrition plans produce stronger results than generic group programs (de Hoogh et al., 2021; Shyam et al., 2022). Tailoring advice to your specific data, needs, and readiness for change leads to actions that stick and results you can measure.

You've learned to advocate for yourself, shape nutrition and activity to fit your life, monitor progress, welcome support, and tackle barriers. Each self-audit and adjustment is one more step toward a confident, lasting relationship with your body and health.

Real success comes from blending proven science with personal wisdom, championing your needs, and refusing to see adaptation as defeat. Mastery isn't perfection; it's steady, curious improvement.

Practical Next Steps

As you move forward, consider these actions:

- **Within the next week:** Schedule a check-in with your provider to discuss long-term goals. Review your current routine and identify one area for adjustment.
- **Within the next month:** Complete a full self-audit using the questions above. Update at least one aspect of your support team, whether that's finding a new online community, reconnecting with a friend for accountability, or scheduling a dietitian consultation.
- **Within the next three months:** Establish a regular rhythm for monitoring trends and making small course corrections. Build sustainable systems that don't require constant willpower.
- **Long-term:** Commit to annual reviews of your blueprint. As treatments evolve and your life changes, your approach should evolve too. Stay curious about new research, new tools, and new ways to support your health.

The landscape of weight management and metabolic health is changing rapidly. Staying informed and flexible positions you to take advantage of new developments while maintaining the foundation you've built.

Your journey with GLP-1s isn't about reaching a finish line where you're "done." It's about building a sustainable way of living that supports your health through all of life's seasons and changes. The tools, strategies, and mindset you've developed throughout this book give you everything needed to navigate whatever comes next.

Conclusion

If you've made it this far, you've committed time, energy, and heart to understanding your body and giving yourself another chance. That's not small. That's huge.

Looking back through these chapters, we've covered a lot of ground together. We started with the science behind GLP-1 medications, how they work in your body, and why they're different from every diet you've tried before. We walked through getting started with therapy, navigating the medical system, and dealing with insurance obstacles that shouldn't exist but do. We talked about practical nutrition strategies, managing side effects, building sustainable habits for busy lives, and overcoming the inevitable plateaus and setbacks.

But more than information, I hope you've gained something deeper: permission. Permission to use medical tools without shame. Permission to prioritize your health. Permission to ask for help. Permission to adapt and change course when something isn't working. And most importantly, permission to be imperfect while still making progress.

What You've Learned

- **Lasting weight loss is achievable:** Not easy, not quick, not without effort, but genuinely possible. Progress may slow, stall, or look different from what you expect. The scale might frustrate you. Old habits might try to resurface. But with the right tools and support, you can build something that lasts.
- **You are allowed to advocate for yourself:** With your provider, with insurance companies, with anyone who doubts you or dismisses your struggles. Your health is worth fighting for. Bring your research to appointments. Ask pointed questions. Push back when you're handed outdated advice. Challenge denials. Keep detailed records. You don't need permission to take up space in your own healthcare.

- **Progress is bigger than the scale:** More energy to play with your kids. Climbing stairs without getting winded. Better lab results. Reduced medication. Improved sleep. Clearer thinking. Greater mobility. These victories are just as real as pounds lost, sometimes more so. Track them. Celebrate them. Let them fuel you when the scale won't budge.
- **Side effects are manageable:** Nausea, fatigue, headaches, constipation, and taste changes are uncomfortable but temporary for most people. You now have strategies: hydration protocols, meal timing techniques, fiber targets, and safe supplements. You know when to push through and when to call your provider. You're not helpless against side effects.
- **Community matters:** You are not alone in this. Millions are walking this same road. Online support groups, local walking buddies, and healthcare teams who actually listen, these connections make the difference between giving up and pushing through. Find your people. Share your struggles and wins. Let others support you, and support them in return.
- **Flexibility beats rigidity:** All-or-nothing thinking is the enemy of long-term success. The ability to adapt, to course-correct without guilt, to try new approaches when old ones stop working, that's where real strength lives. Your blueprint isn't set in stone. It evolves with you.

The real message I really want you to take away from this book is that your body is not broken. Your struggles with weight aren't personal failings or a lack of willpower. They're biological challenges that can be overcome with the right tools and support.

You now hold a blueprint, not just mine, but yours, for lasting change. You have the science. You have the strategies. You have permission to use medical help without shame. You have a roadmap for navigating obstacles.

What you do with all of this is up to you.

The tools are yours now. The knowledge is yours. And most importantly, the power to change your story is yours.

I believe in your ability to succeed, not because success is guaranteed, but because you're willing to keep showing up. That's the only requirement that really matters.

So here's to your next chapter. To better health, more energy, less pain, greater mobility, and the freedom that comes from knowing you have control over your own body and choices.

Here's to progress over perfection.

Here's to consistency over intensity.

Here's to grace over guilt.

Here's to you.

You've got this. Now go build the life you deserve.

***

P.S. If you found value in this book, please consider sharing your story in online communities. Your experience, your struggles, your victories, they matter to someone else who's just starting out and needs to know they're not alone. We rise by lifting others. Be part of that rising.

Help Me By Leaving A Review

I hope The GLP-1 Weight Loss Blueprint leads you to a new path, one that helps you feel stronger, healthier, and more at ease with your body. Writing this book was a journey of learning and growth for me, and I'm grateful that you chose to be part of it.

If you enjoyed what you read, leaving a short review on Amazon makes a real difference. Your feedback helps others discover the book and encourages me to keep creating work that supports happier, more sustainable living.

Thank you for supporting independent authors and for choosing to invest in your well-being. It means more than you know.

Keep learning, keep growing, and stay kind to the person you are becoming.

To leave a review:

• Scan the QR code provided in this book

• Or search for the title on Amazon, open the book page, and click where the next to where Star ratings are, then click

Write a Customer Review.

Glossary

A1C (HbA1c): A blood test that measures average blood sugar levels over the past two to three months, used to diagnose and monitor diabetes and prediabetes. Even a 1% reduction in A1C can lower the risk of diabetes complications by up to 30%.

Adaptive thermogenesis: The slowdown in metabolism and reduction in calories burned as the body adapts to weight loss, often causing plateaus.

All-or-nothing thinking: A rigid mindset where one views situations in black-and-white terms, such as being either perfectly on track or completely off track, which undermines long-term success.

Appetite suppression: The primary effect of GLP-1 medications, reducing hunger signals and food cravings to make eating less feel more natural.

Batch cooking/meal prep: Preparing multiple meals or meal components at once (typically on weekends) to ensure healthy options are readily available throughout busy weeks.

Behavioral drift: The gradual return of old habits, such as increased portion sizes or less physical activity, which can stall weight loss progress.

Blood sugar (glucose): The concentration of glucose in the blood, which is a primary source of energy for the body's cells and is regulated by insulin and other hormones.

Bloating: A feeling of fullness, tightness, or swelling in the abdomen, often caused by slowed digestion or gas buildup, common with GLP-1 medications.

Bluetooth-enabled scale: A digital scale that syncs weight and body composition data to apps like Apple Health or MyFitnessPal for trend monitoring over time.

BMI (body mass index): A measure of body fat based on height and weight, often used by insurance companies as criteria for medication approval, though it has limitations.

Body composition: The percentages of fat, muscle, bone, and water in the body, which smart scales can measure beyond simple weight.

Chronic pain: Long-lasting pain that persists beyond the usual recovery period or accompanies a chronic health condition, which can affect metabolism, mobility, and weight management.

Cognitive restructuring: A therapeutic technique to identify and change negative thought patterns, often used to combat self-criticism and internalized weight bias.

Compounded medications: Custom-made medications prepared by specialty pharmacies when brand-name drugs are unavailable or unaffordable; they typically cost $200-400 monthly but may have variable quality and lack FDA oversight.

Compounding pharmacy: A specialty pharmacy that creates custom formulations of medications, sometimes used as a more affordable alternative to brand-name GLP-1s.

Constipation: Difficulty or infrequency in bowel movements, a common side effect of GLP-1 medications due to slowed gastric emptying; manageable with fiber, hydration, and movement.

Continuous glucose monitors (CGMs): Wearable devices like Dexcom G7 or FreeStyle Libre that track blood glucose levels in real-time, providing feedback on how foods and activities affect blood sugar.

Cortisol: A hormone released in response to stress that can affect metabolism, inflammation, sleep, and weight gain, particularly problematic in chronic pain conditions.

Dehydration signs: Symptoms such as extreme thirst, dark urine, dizziness when standing, rapid heartbeat, and confusion indicating insufficient fluid intake.

Delayed gastric emptying: A common effect of GLP-1 medications, where food moves more slowly from the stomach to the small intestine, causing prolonged fullness and potential constipation.

Dexcom/FreeStyle Libre: Specific brands of continuous glucose monitors that sync with smartphones to track blood sugar patterns throughout the day.

Diet culture: A societal system that equates thinness with health and moral virtue, often promoting restrictive dieting at any cost and blaming individuals for weight issues rather than recognizing biological factors.

Diet fatigue: Emotional and physical exhaustion resulting from repeated cycles of dieting, restriction, and weight loss attempts without lasting success.

Digital health tools: Apps, smartwatches, and connected devices that support tracking of diet, activity, weight, and health metrics to provide data-driven insights.

Digital medication reminders: Apps like Medisafe and alarm systems that help patients remember dosing schedules for medications like weekly GLP-1 injections.

Dose escalation: The gradual increase in medication dosage over time, synonymous with titration, designed to minimize side effects while finding the optimal therapeutic dose.

Dual agonists: Newer medications like tirzepatide that target multiple hormone receptors (GLP-1 and GIP) simultaneously to enhance weight loss and metabolic control beyond single-action drugs.

Electrolyte balance: The proper levels of minerals like sodium, potassium, and magnesium necessary for hydration, muscle function, and preventing side effects like headaches and fatigue.

Electrolyte drinks: Low-sugar beverages like LMNT, Nuun, or Pedialyte that help maintain hydration and mineral balance, particularly useful for managing GLP-1 side effects.

Emergency kit: A portable collection of supplies for managing symptoms on-the-go, such as ginger chews, protein snacks, acupressure bands, and disposable bags for nausea.

Emotional eating: Eating triggered by stress, boredom, anxiety, or habit rather than genuine physical hunger; GLP-1s primarily address physical hunger but not emotional eating patterns.

Energy window: The time of day when an individual has the highest energy levels and lowest pain, optimal for scheduling physical activity and movement.

Fatigue: Overwhelming tiredness and lack of energy, one of the common early side effects of GLP-1 medications that typically improves within 2-4 weeks.

Food aversion: A decreased desire for or negative reaction to certain foods, often experienced during GLP-1 treatment, particularly toward greasy, sweet, or rich items.

Food fatigue: Getting tired of eating the same foods repeatedly, which can be addressed by rotating meal options and using herbs and spices for variety.

Food noise: The constant mental chatter and intrusive thoughts about food, cravings, meal planning, and what to eat next, which GLP-1s help quiet significantly.

Gallbladder problems/gallstones: Potential serious complications with GLP-1 use that require medical attention, especially if experiencing severe upper right abdominal pain with fever.

Gastric emptying: The process by which food moves from the stomach to the small intestine, which GLP-1 medications deliberately slow to promote satiety.

Gastrointestinal (GI) side effects: Symptoms like nausea, constipation, bloating, gas, and reflux caused by GLP-1 medications' effects on the digestive system.

Ghrelin: Known as the "hunger hormone," it is produced in the stomach and signals hunger to the brain. Levels can rise 20-25% after weight loss, intensifying appetite.

GIP receptor: A hormone receptor targeted alongside GLP-1 by dual-action medications like tirzepatide to improve weight loss and blood sugar control.

GLP-1 (Glucagon-like peptide-1): A naturally occurring hormone produced in the intestines and brain that regulates appetite, blood sugar, and digestion; targeted by certain medications to aid weight loss and metabolic health.

GLP-1 therapies: Prescription medications that mimic or enhance natural GLP-1 to help regulate hunger, satiety, and blood sugar control for weight management and diabetes treatment.

Glucagon: A hormone that signals the liver to release stored glucose into the bloodstream; GLP-1 medications suppress inappropriate glucagon release to prevent blood sugar spikes.

Gut-brain axis/signaling: The communication system between the digestive tract and brain that regulates hunger, fullness, and food reward; altered by GLP-1 medications to reduce appetite.

Habit stacking: A behavior change technique where new habits are linked to existing routines, such as doing calf raises while brushing teeth or squats during commercial breaks.

Hair loss: A rare but possible side effect of rapid weight loss on GLP-1 medications, often related to nutritional deficiencies that can be prevented with adequate protein intake.

Headaches: Tension-type headaches across the forehead or neck, one of the common early side effects of GLP-1s, typically improving within one to two weeks and manageable with hydration.

Healthcare provider: A medical professional such as a doctor, nurse practitioner, or physician assistant who diagnoses conditions, manages patient care, and prescribes and monitors medications.

Health markers: Measurable indicators of health such as blood pressure, cholesterol levels, blood sugar, inflammation markers, and liver function that often improve with GLP-1 therapy.

Hydration protocols/strategies: Techniques like steady water intake (8-10 cups daily), electrolyte supplementation, and setting phone reminders to manage side effects and support overall health.

Hypothalamus: A small, almond-sized region deep in the brain that acts as the control center for hunger, appetite, satiety signals, and weight regulation.

Inflammation: A chronic condition that contributes to pain and metabolic dysfunction; reduced through weight loss, with every pound lost relieving approximately 4 pounds of pressure from joints.

Insulin: A hormone that helps cells absorb glucose from the bloodstream; GLP-1s enhance insulin release in response to meals while preventing dangerous low blood sugar.

Insulin resistance: A condition where cells respond poorly to insulin, leading to higher insulin levels, increased fat storage, and difficulty losing weight, often improved with GLP-1 therapy.

Insurance approval: The process by which an insurance company authorizes coverage for a prescribed medication or treatment, often requiring prior authorization and documentation.

Internalized weight stigma: When a person absorbs negative societal attitudes about weight and applies them to themselves, damaging self-esteem, motivation, and mental health.

Leptin: A hormone produced by fat cells that signals fullness to the brain. Leptin levels drop after fat loss, weakening satiety signals and making weight maintenance more difficult.

Letter of medical necessity: A formal document from a healthcare provider explaining why a specific treatment is essential for a patient's health, used in insurance appeals.

Liraglutide: The active ingredient in Victoza and Saxenda, a GLP-1 medication requiring daily injections but with extensive long-term safety data.

LMNT: A specific brand of electrolyte drink mix with no sugar, frequently recommended for managing hydration and preventing headaches on GLP-1s.

Manufacturer savings programs: Financial assistance programs offered by pharmaceutical companies to reduce copays for commercially insured patients, often reducing costs to $25-150 monthly.

Meal planning: Structuring meals and snacks in advance to ensure adequate nutrition and protein intake, especially important when appetite is significantly reduced.

Meal timing modification: Adjusting when meals are eaten to better align with natural appetite patterns, energy levels, and metabolic responses on GLP-1 medications.

Medical history: A comprehensive record of a patient's past health information, including conditions, treatments, medications, lab results, and previous weight loss attempts.

Medical necessity: A term used by insurers to describe treatments deemed essential for a patient's health and qualifying for coverage, requiring documentation to prove.

Medication adherence: The degree to which a patient correctly follows prescribed medication schedules, doses, and instructions for optimal results.

Medication storage: Proper handling and temperature control of GLP-1 medications (refrigeration at home, insulated pouches with ice packs when traveling) to maintain effectiveness.

Medication titration: Gradual dose increases of a medication over time, typically every two to four weeks, to minimize side effects and find the optimal therapeutic dose for each individual.

Metabolic adaptation: A slowdown in metabolism and increased energy efficiency that occurs after weight loss, making further weight loss difficult and maintenance challenging.

Metabolic resistance: The body's biological response to calorie restriction, where metabolism slows down and hunger hormones increase to conserve energy and restore lost weight.

Metabolism: The chemical processes in the body that convert food into energy; it naturally slows with age, weight loss, and chronic dieting.

Mounjaro: Brand name for tirzepatide when prescribed for type 2 diabetes management, a dual GLP-1/GIP agonist showing enhanced weight loss compared to single-action medications.

Multi-hormone receptor agonists: Drugs like triple agonists currently in development that activate several hormonal pathways simultaneously to produce greater therapeutic effects.

Nausea: The most common early side effect of GLP-1 medications, typically peaking two to six hours after injection, lasting one to three days, and improving significantly after two to three weeks.

Neurobiology: The study of the nervous system, including brain regions like the hypothalamus, ventral tegmental area, and nucleus accumbens that influence hunger, reward, cravings, and eating behavior.

Non-responder: A person who experiences little to no appetite suppression or weight loss after several months of consistent, appropriately dosed GLP-1 use; genuinely rare, occurring in a small percentage of users.

Non-scale victories (NSVs): Positive outcomes in health and well-being not reflected on the scale, such as improved energy, better sleep, reduced pain, lower blood pressure, enhanced mobility, or improved mood.

Nutrient density: The concentration of essential nutrients (vitamins, minerals, protein, healthy fats) per calorie in foods; critically important to focus on when eating significantly smaller portions.

Off-label prescribing: The legal and common practice of doctors prescribing medications for purposes not specifically FDA-approved, such as Ozempic for weight loss in non-diabetic patients.

Oral GLP-1 medications: Pills like Rybelsus that deliver GLP-1 receptor agonists, potentially improving convenience versus injections but requiring strict dosing conditions (empty stomach, 30-minute wait before eating).

Over-the-counter (OTC) remedies: Non-prescription options like acetaminophen for headaches, magnesium supplements, polyethylene glycol (MiraLAX), fiber gummies, or stool softeners to manage side effects.

Ozempic: Brand name for semaglutide specifically approved for type 2 diabetes management but frequently prescribed off-label for weight loss, dosed up to 2 mg weekly.

Pancreatitis: A serious potential complication involving inflammation of the pancreas, requiring immediate medical attention if experiencing severe abdominal pain with fever, nausea, and vomiting.

Patient assistance programs: Financial aid programs for uninsured or underinsured patients who meet income requirements, sometimes providing free or heavily discounted medications.

PCOS (Polycystic Ovary Syndrome): A hormonal condition affecting metabolism and weight, often benefiting from GLP-1 therapy through improved insulin sensitivity and reduced inflammation.

Pedialyte: An electrolyte replacement drink originally designed for children but useful for adults managing dehydration and maintaining mineral balance on GLP-1s.

Peer-to-peer review: An insurance appeals process where a physician reviews a patient's case with the insurance company's medical reviewer to argue for coverage approval.

Perfectionism: An all-or-nothing mindset that sets unrealistic standards and interprets any deviation as failure, undermining long-term success and requiring cognitive restructuring.

Perimenopause: The transitional phase before menopause, characterized by hormonal fluctuations (particularly estrogen) affecting metabolism, gut function, sleep, mood, and weight management.

Physical hunger: The biological need for food, signaled gradually by the body (slight stomach pressure, fatigue) and satisfied by various foods; GLP-1s primarily affect this type of hunger.

Plateau: A period during weight loss, typically 3+ weeks, where progress stalls despite continued consistent efforts, often due to adaptive thermogenesis and metabolic adaptation.

Portion control: Eating appropriate amounts based on new hunger and fullness cues rather than external portion sizes, using strategies like smaller plates and the "palm of hand" measurement for protein.

Prediabetes: A condition where blood sugar levels are elevated (A1C 5.7-6.4%) but not yet in the diabetic range, often improved or reversed with GLP-1 therapy and lifestyle changes.

Prior authorization: An insurance process requiring approval before coverage of certain medications, typically involving submission of medical necessity documentation and proof of failed conservative treatments.

Progress tracking: Monitoring various health and behavioral metrics over time using apps, journals, or wearables to assess changes beyond just weight, including energy, mood, sleep, and activity.

Protein distribution: Spreading protein intake evenly throughout the day (20-30 grams per meal) rather than loading it all at one meal, which better supports muscle maintenance and provides sustained energy.

Protein power/targets: Emphasizing adequate protein intake of approximately 1.0-1.2 grams per kilogram of body weight daily (75-88 grams for a 160-pound person) to support muscle maintenance, blood sugar stability, and satiety during weight loss.

Psychological barriers: Mental or emotional obstacles that interfere with wellness behaviors, such as fear of judgment at gyms, past negative experiences, or internalized shame about weight.

Rebound effect: The potential for rapid weight regain or intensified side effects when discontinuing or reducing GLP-1 medication too quickly without proper tapering protocols.

Reflux/heartburn: Burning sensation in the chest or throat when stomach acid backs up, sometimes occurring with GLP-1s and manageable by avoiding trigger foods, staying upright after meals, and elevating the head of the bed.

Relapse prevention: Strategies to maintain weight loss and healthy habits while avoiding setbacks, including regular monitoring, early intervention protocols, maintaining support systems, and having emergency meal plans.

Reset meals: Simple, bland, easy-to-digest meals for difficult days when appetite is very low or nausea is present, such as soft scrambled eggs with toast, plain rice with vegetables, or chicken broth.

Reward pathways: Brain circuits involving the ventral tegmental area and nucleus accumbens that determine what's rewarding and drive food-seeking behavior; modulated by GLP-1 medications to reduce food cravings.

Rybelsus: The oral (pill) form of semaglutide requiring specific dosing conditions—taken on an empty stomach first thing in the morning with minimal water, then waiting 30 minutes before eating or drinking.

Satiety: The feeling of fullness, satisfaction, and lack of desire to eat more after consuming food; enhanced significantly by GLP-1 medications through multiple mechanisms.

Self-advocacy: Actively participating in one's healthcare by preparing documentation, communicating needs clearly, asking informed questions, challenging dismissive advice, and pushing back against insurance denials.

Self-compassion: Treating oneself with kindness, understanding, and patience during trials and setbacks rather than harsh self-criticism; shown to support lasting change better than self-judgment.

Semaglutide: A GLP-1 receptor agonist used in medications like Ozempic (diabetes), Wegovy (weight loss), and Rybelsus (oral diabetes) to regulate appetite and blood sugar.

Set-point theory: The concept that the body defends a certain weight range through physiological mechanisms (metabolic adaptation, hormone changes) to maintain stability, like a thermostat.

Step therapy: An insurance policy requiring patients to try less expensive treatments (like metformin or lifestyle modification) before coverage is approved for more costly drugs like GLP-1s.

Stress-pain-weight connection: The interplay where chronic pain increases stress hormones (cortisol), promotes inflammation, disrupts sleep quality, and reduces mobility, all contributing to weight gain and making weight loss more difficult.

Tapering GLP-1 medication: Gradually reducing dosage under medical supervision over several months to maintain results, minimize rebound effects, and assess ability to maintain weight independently.

Taste changes: Alterations in how foods taste or smell, a common side effect where previously enjoyed foods (especially greasy, sweet, or rich items) become unappealing during GLP-1 treatment.

Technology overwhelm: Feeling stressed, burdened, or fatigued by too many health tracking devices, apps, or notifications; manageable by simplifying to one to two key metrics and muting non-essential alerts.

Telemedicine: The remote delivery of healthcare services and consultations via digital technologies, increasingly used for GLP-1 prescribing and follow-up care.

Thyroid issues: Conditions like hypothyroidism or Hashimoto's that affect metabolism and can slow weight loss, requiring screening and treatment alongside GLP-1 therapy.

Tirzepatide: A dual-action medication targeting both GLP-1 and GIP receptors to enhance weight loss (16-21% body weight) and blood sugar control beyond single-action medications, sold as Mounjaro (diabetes) and Zepbound (weight loss).

Trulicity (dulaglutide): A weekly injection GLP-1 medication that some people tolerate better than semaglutide options, offering similar benefits with potentially fewer side effects for sensitive individuals.

Type 2 diabetes: A chronic condition characterized by high blood sugar and insulin resistance, for which many GLP-1 medications were originally developed and remain highly effective treatments.

Victoza (liraglutide): A daily injection GLP-1 medication with extensive long-term safety data, used primarily for diabetes management but also available as Saxenda for weight loss.

Wegovy: Brand-name semaglutide specifically approved for weight management with dosing up to 2.4 mg weekly, higher than Ozempic, and specifically FDA-approved for adolescents 12+ meeting criteria.

Weight cycling: The repeated pattern of losing weight and regaining it (often called yo-yo dieting), which can worsen metabolic adaptation and make future weight loss more difficult.

Weight loss stigma: Social and cultural biases, judgment, and discrimination against people with overweight or obesity, which can affect mental health, treatment-seeking behavior, and healthcare quality.

Weight loss supplements: Non-prescription products claiming to aid weight loss, typically lacking scientific validation, FDA oversight, or endorsement by medical organizations; distinguished from prescription GLP-1 medications.

Weight regain: The return of lost weight after dieting or weight loss attempts, often due to biological factors (increased ghrelin, decreased leptin, metabolic adaptation) rather than lack of willpower.

Yo-yo dieting: Popular term for weight cycling—the repeated pattern of losing and regaining weight through successive diet attempts, which can damage metabolism and mental health over time.

Zepbound: Brand name for tirzepatide when specifically prescribed for weight loss rather than diabetes management, with the same dual GLP-1/GIP mechanism as Mounjaro.

References

Abeltino, A., Riente, A., Bianchetti, G., Serantoni, C., Spirito, M. D., Capezzone, S., Esposito, R., & Maulucci, G. (2024). Digital applications for diet monitoring, planning, and precision nutrition for citizens and professionals: a state of the art. *Nutrition Reviews, 83*(2). https://doi.org/10.1093/nutrit/nuae035

Adkison, J. (2022, August 18). *Comparing ozempic, wegovy and other GLP-1 drugs*. GoodRx. https://www.goodrx.com/classes/glp-1-agonists/glp-1-drugs-comparison?srsltid=AfmBOoqzHPO89_VZANC1lJR3z3phS6pIZNDONDFL7v3gakDnYCicctsS

Aghajanian, C., Bell-McGuinn, K. M., Burris, H. A., Siu, L. L., Stayner, L.-A., Wheler, J. J., Hong, D. S., Kurkjian, C., Pant, S., Santiago-Walker, A., Gauvin, J. L., Antal, J. M., Opalinska, J. B., Morris, S. R., & Infante, J. R. (2018). A phase I, open-label, two-stage study to investigate the safety, tolerability, pharmacokinetics, and pharmacodynamics of the oral AKT inhibitor GSK2141795 in patients with solid tumors. *Investigational New Drugs, 36*(6), 1016–1025. https://doi.org/10.1007/s10637-018-0591-z

American Diabetes Association. (2024, December 2). *The American Diabetes Association announces statement on compounded incretin products*. https://diabetes.org/newsroom/press-releases/american-diabetes-association-announces-statement-compounded-incretin

American Psychological Association. (2012, January 26). *What you need to know about willpower: The psychological science of self-control.* https://www.apa.org/topics/personality/willpower

Amorim, G., Teranishi, M., Claudia, A., James, F., & Perera, S. (2025). Mechanisms of GLP-1 in modulating craving and addiction: Neurobiological and translational insights. *Medical Sciences*, *13*(3), 136–136. https://doi.org/10.3390/medsci13030136

Anderson, S. L., & Marrs, J. C. (2023). Tirzepatide for type 2 diabetes. *Drugs in Context*, *12*, 1–8. https://doi.org/10.7573/dic.2023-6-1

Avcilar, T. (2022). ZoomForward2022: European Congress on obesity. *Obesity Facts*, *15*(Suppl. 1), 1–240. https://doi.org/10.1159/000524469

Bertagna, B. (2024, May 22). *9 steps to appeal A prior authorization denial for weight loss meds*. Klarity Health, Inc. https://www.helloklarity.com/post/appeal-prior-authorization-denial/

Borja, R. (2020, December 18). *6 weight loss myths — and what really works to drop pounds*. AARP. https://www.aarp.org/health/healthy-living/weight-loss-myths/

Billingsley, A. (2022, December 7). *Wegovy vs. Ozempic: How are they different?* GoodRx. https://www.goodrx.com/classes/glp-1-agonists/wegovy-vs-ozempic?srsltid=AfmBOoo_ftGmKGLPh1ipPS31EeE4WgJdwAEoxzNxSKUrq94ruNnCQokh

Capehorn, M., Ghani, Y., Hindsberger, C., Johansen, P., & Jódar, E. (2020). Once-Weekly semaglutide reduces HbA1c and body weight in patients with type 2 diabetes regardless of background common OAD: A subgroup analysis from SUSTAIN 2–4 and 10. *Diabetes Therapy*, *11*(5), 1061–1075. https://doi.org/10.1007/s13300-020-00796-z

Chappell, A. (2025, March 19). *Why high insulin levels make you crave carbs and sugar and how to fix it.* Lilli Health. https://lillihealth.com/why-high-insulin-levels-make-you-crave-carbs-and-sugar-and-how-to-fix-it/

Chesak, J. (2025, May 19). *Ozempic constipation: How to treat it and prevent another bout.* Oshi Health. https://oshihealth.com/ozempic-constipation/

Ciampolini, M., Lovell-Smith, Bianchi, & Kenealy, T. (2013). Hunger can be taught: Hunger recognition regulates eating and improves energy balance. *International Journal of General Medicine, 6*, 465. https://doi.org/10.2147/ijgm.s40655

Conley, M. (2025, April 1). *Five things to know about GLP-1s and addiction.* Stanford Medicine News Center. https://med.stanford.edu/news/insights/2025/04/ozempic-addiction-glp-1s-mounjaro-lembke.html

Considering GLP-1 medications? What they are and why lifestyle change is key to sustained weight loss. (2023, August 22). *Mayo Clinic Diet.* https://diet.mayoclinic.org/us/blog/2023/considering-glp-1-medications-what-they-are-and-why-lifestyle-change-is-key-to-sustained-weight-loss/

Contreras, F., Al-Najim, W., & le Roux, C. W. (2024). Health benefits beyond the scale: The role of diet and nutrition during weight loss programmes. *Nutrients, 16*(21), 3585. https://doi.org/10.3390/nu16213585

Dailey, M. J., & Moran, T. H. (2013). Glucagon-like peptide 1 and appetite. *Trends in Endocrinology & Metabolism, 24*(2), 85–91. https://doi.org/10.1016/j.tem.2012.11.008

Davies, S. W., Putnam, H. M., Ainsworth, T., Baum, J. K., Bove, C. B., Crosby, S. C., Côté, I. M., Duplouy, A., Fulweiler, R. W., Griffin, A. J., Hanley, T. C., Hill, T., Humanes, A., Mangubhai, S., Metaxas, A., Parker, L. M., Rivera, H. E., Silbiger, N. J., Smith, N. S., & Spalding, A. K. (2021). Promoting inclusive metrics of success and impact to dismantle a discriminatory reward system in science. *PLOS Biology, 19*(6), e3001282. https://doi.org/10.1371/journal.pbio.3001282

de Hoogh, I. M., Winters, B. L., Nieman, K. M., Bijlsma, S., Krone, T., van den Broek, T. J., Anderson, B. D., Caspers, M. P. M., Anthony, J. C., & Wopereis, S. (2021). A novel personalized systems nutrition program improves dietary patterns, lifestyle behaviors and health-related outcomes: Results from the habit study. *Nutrients*, *13*(6), 1763. https://doi.org/10.3390/nu13061763

Dodier, S. (2024, October 28). *Achievable goals post-diet culture: Clean vs dirty goals*. Going beyond the Food. https://www.stephaniedodier.com/achievable-goals-post-diet-culture/

Drugs.com. (2025, October 17). *Tirzepatide vs semaglutide: How do they compare?* Drugs.com. https://www.drugs.com/medical-answers/tirzepatide-semaglutide-how-compare-3576410/

Eli Lilly and Company. (2025, September 17). *Lilly's Mounjaro (tirzepatide), a GIP/GLP-1 dual receptor agonist, reduced A1C by an average of 2.2% in a Phase 3 trial of children and adolescents with type 2 diabetes*. Cision PR Newswire. https://www.prnewswire.com/news-releases/lillys-mounjaro-tirzepatide-a-gipglp-1-dual-receptor-agonist-reduced-a1c-by-an-average-of-2-2-in-a-phase-3-trial-of-children-and-adolescents-with-type-2-diabetes-302559576.html

Fitch, A., Gigliotti, L., & Bays, H. E. (2025). Application of nutrition interventions with GLP-1 based therapies: A narrative review of the challenges and solutions. *Obesity Pillars*, *16*, 100205. https://doi.org/10.1016/j.obpill.2025.100205

Fothergill, E., Guo, J., Howard, L., Kerns, J. C., Knuth, N. D., Brychta, R., Chen, K. Y., Skarulis, M. C., Walter, M., Walter, P. J., & Hall, K. D. (2016). Persistent metabolic adaptation 6 years after "The Biggest Loser" competition. *Obesity*, *24*(8), 1612–1619. https://doi.org/10.1002/oby.21538

Frequently asked questions: OPTAVIA lifestyle program to support GLP-1s. (2025, July 8). Optavia. https://coachanswers.optavia.com/help/s/article/Frequently-Asked-Questions-OPTAVIA-Lifestyle-Program-to-Support-GLP-1s?language=en_US

García-Gorrita, C., San Onofre, N., Merino-Torres, J. F., & Soriano, J. M. (2025). Beyond GLP-1 agonists: An adaptive ketogenic–mediterranean protocol to counter metabolic adaptation in obesity management. *Nutrients, 17*(16), 2699. https://doi.org/10.3390/nu17162699

Hall, K. D. (2023). Physiology of the weight loss plateau after calorie restriction, GLP-1 receptor agonism, and bariatric surgery. *BioRxiv (Cold Spring Harbor Laboratory).* https://doi.org/10.1101/2023.11.05.565699

Hall, K. D., & Kahan, S. (2018). Maintenance of lost weight and long-term management of obesity. *Medical Clinics of North America, 102*(1), 183–197. https://doi.org/10.1016/j.mcna.2017.08.012

Hansen, T. K., Dall, R., Hosoda, H., Kojima, M., Kangawa, K., Christiansen, J. S., & Jorgensen, J. O. L. (2002). Weight loss increases circulating levels of ghrelin in human obesity. *Clinical Endocrinology, 56*(2), 203–206. https://doi.org/10.1046/j.0300-0664.2001.01456.x

Health 360. (2025, March 19). *Your friendly guide to GLP-1 weight loss: what works, what doesn't and what's next.* Intermountain Healthcare. https://intermountainhealthcare.org/blogs/your-friendly-guide-to-glp-1-weight-loss-what-works-what-doesnt-and-whats-next

Hosseini, M. M., Hosseini, S. T. M., Qayumi, K., Hosseinzadeh, S., & Tabar, S. S. S. (2023). Smartwatches in healthcare medicine: Assistance and monitoring; a Scoping review. *BMC Medical Informatics and Decision Making, 23*(1), 248. https://doi.org/10.1186/s12911-023-02350-w

The importance of weight management. (2025, April 11). Information Site. https://mydiabetesmyway.scot.nhs.uk/resources/internal/the-importance-of-weight-management/

Improving the patient onboarding experience and reducing scale support time for a virtual medical weight loss program. (2024, February 1). Withings Health Solutions. https://withingshealthsolutions.com/improving-patient-onboarding-experience-and-reducing-scale-support-time-for-virtual-medical-weight-loss-program/

Jastreboff, A. M., Sinha, R., Lacadie, C., Small, D. M., Sherwin, R. S., & Potenza, M. N. (2013). Neural correlates of stress- and food cue–induced food craving in obesity: Association with insulin levels. *Diabetes Care, 36*(2), 394–402. https://doi.org/10.2337/dc12-1112

Keeping track of your success without obsessing over the scale. (2022, December 1). Garnet Health. https://www.garnethealth.org/news/keeping-track-your-success-without-obsessing-over-scale

Keesey, R. E., & Hirvonen, M. D. (1997). Body weight set-points: Determination and adjustment. *The Journal of Nutrition, 127*(9), 1875S1883S. https://doi.org/10.1093/jn/127.9.1875s

Knerr, P. J., Mowery, S. A., Douros, J. D., Premdjee, B., Hjøllund, K., R., He, Y., Hansen, A., K., Olsen, A., Perez-Tilve, D., DiMarchi, R. D., & Finan, B. (2022). Next generation GLP-1/GIP/glucagon triple agonists normalize body weight in obese mice. *Molecular Metabolism, 63*, 101533–101533. https://doi.org/10.1016/j.molmet.2022.101533

Kumar, R. B., & Aronne, L. J. (2024, August 20). *Pharmacologic treatment of obesity.* South Dartmouth (MA): MDText.com, Inc. https://www.ncbi.nlm.nih.gov/books/NBK279038/

Latif, W., Lambrinos, K. J., & Rodriguez, R. (2024, February 25). *Compare and contrast the glucagon-like peptide-1 receptor agonists (GLP-1Ras)*. PubMed; StatPearls Publishing. https://www.ncbi.nlm.nih.gov/books/NBK572151/

Lau, E. Y., Mitchell, M. S., & Faulkner, G. (2022). Long-term usage of a commercial mHealth app: A "multiple-lives" perspective. *Frontiers in Public Health, 10*. https://doi.org/10.3389/fpubh.2022.914433

Leptin: What it is, function, levels & leptin resistance. (2022, March 3). Cleveland Clinic. https://my.clevelandclinic.org/health/body/22446-leptin

Lonnie, M., Hooker, E., Brunstrom, J., Corfe, B., Green, M., Watson, A., Williams, E., Stevenson, E., Penson, S., & Johnstone, A. (2018). Protein for life: Review of optimal protein intake, sustainable dietary sources and the effect on appetite in ageing Adults. *Nutrients, 10*(3), 360. https://doi.org/10.3390/nu10030360

Mamerow, M. M., Mettler, J. A., English, K. L., Casperson, S. L., Arentson-Lantz, E., Sheffield-Moore, M., Layman, D. K., & Paddon-Jones, D. (2014). Dietary protein distribution positively influences 24-h muscle protein synthesis in healthy adults. *The Journal of Nutrition, 144*(6), 876–880. https://doi.org/10.3945/jn.113.185280

Managing weight with Wegovy. (n.d.). Wegovy. https://www.wegovy.com/about-wegovy/managing-weight-with-wegovy.html

Mawer, R. (2023, December 21). *Ghrelin: The "hunger hormone" explained.* Healthline. https://www.healthline.com/nutrition/ghrelin

Mayo Clinic Staff. (2023, August 26). *Exercise: 7 benefits of regular physical activity.* Mayo Clinic. https://www.mayoclinic.org/healthy-lifestyle/fitness/in-depth/exercise/art-20048389

Mayo Clinic Staff. (2025, September 19). *Exercise and stress: Get moving to manage stress*. Mayo Clinic. https://www.mayoclinic.org/healthy-lifestyle/stress-management/in-depth/exercise-and-stress/art-20044469

Messier, S. P., Gutekunst, D. J., Davis, C., & DeVita, P. (2005). Weight loss reduces knee-joint loads in overweight and obese older adults with knee osteoarthritis. *Arthritis & Rheumatism, 52*(7), 2026–2032. https://doi.org/10.1002/art.21139

Mozaffarian, D., Agarwal, M., Aggarwal, M., Alexander, L., Apovian, C. M., Bindlish, S., Bonnet, J., Butsch, W. S., Christensen, S., Gianos, E., Gulati, M., Gupta, A., Horn, D., Kane, R. M., Saluja, J., Sannidhi, D., Stanford, F. C., & Callahan, E. A. (2025). Nutritional priorities to support GLP-1 therapy for obesity: a joint Advisory from the American College of Lifestyle Medicine, the American Society for Nutrition, the Obesity Medicine Association, and The Obesity Society. *The American Journal of Clinical Nutrition, 122*(1). https://doi.org/10.1016/j.ajcnut.2025.04.023

Mulcahy, J., DeLaRosby, A., & Norwood, T. (2025). Transforming care: Implications of glucagon like peptide-1 receptor agonists on physical therapist practice. *Physical Therapy, 105*(6), pzaf061. https://doi.org/10.1093/ptj/pzaf061

Murray, G., Gottlieb, J., & Swartz, H. A. (2020). Maintaining daily routines to stabilize mood: Theory, data, and potential intervention for circadian consequences of COVID-19. *The Canadian Journal of Psychiatry, 66*(1), 9–13. https://doi.org/10.1177/0706743720957825

New GLP-1 therapies enhance quality of weight loss by improving muscle preservation. (2025, June 23). American Diabetes Association. https://diabetes.org/newsroom/press-releases/new-glp-1-therapies-enhance-quality-weight-loss-improving-muscle-0

Nieuwlaat, R., Wilczynski, N., Navarro, T., Hobson, N., Jeffery, R., Keepanasseril, A., Agoritsas, T., Mistry, N., Iorio, A., Jack, S., Sivaramalingam, B., Iserman, E., Mustafa, R. A., Jedraszewski, D., Cotoi, C., & Haynes, R. B. (2014). Interventions for enhancing medication adherence. *Cochrane Database of Systematic Reviews*, *11*(11). https://doi.org/10.1002/14651858.cd000011.pub4

Niezgoda, N., Chomiuk, T., Kasiak, P., Mamcarz, A., & Śliż, D. (2025). The impact of physical activity on weight loss in relation to the pillars of lifestyle medicine—a narrative review. *Nutrients*, *17*(6), 1095. https://doi.org/10.3390/nu17061095

Noble, D. (2023, December 6). *Habits: why are they so hard to change?*. Mayo Clinic Press. https://mcpress.mayoclinic.org/living-well/habits-why-are-they-so-hard-to-change/

Non scale victories. (n.d.). Mercy Medical Center. https://www.mercycare.org/bhs/health-wellness/wellness-resource-library/non-scale-victories/

Olukorode, J. O., Orimoloye, D. A., Nwachukwu, N. O., Onwuzo, C. N., Oloyede, P. O., Temiloluwa Fayemi, Odunaike, O. S., Ayobami-Ojo, P. S., Divine, N., Alo, D. J., & Alex, C. U. (2024). Recent advances and therapeutic benefits of glucagon-like peptide-1 (GLP-1) agonists in the management of type 2 diabetes and associated metabolic disorders. *Cureus*, *16*(10). https://doi.org/10.7759/cureus.72080

Owens, N. (2025, June 20). *What is a weight loss plateau?* WebMD. https://www.webmd.com/obesity/weight-loss-plateau

Perreault, L., Davies, M., Frias, J. P., Laursen, P. N., Lingvay, I., Machineni, S., Varbo, A., Wilding, J. P. H., Wallenstein, S. O. R., & le Roux, C. W. (2022). Changes in glucose metabolism and glycemic status with once-weekly subcutaneous semaglutide 2.4 mg among participants with prediabetes in the STEP program. *Diabetes Care*, *45*(10). https://doi.org/10.2337/dc21-1785

Philip, S. R., Standen, E. C., Schueler, J., Fields, S. A., & Phelan, S. M. (2025). Weight bias in mental health settings: a scoping review. *Frontiers in Psychiatry, 16*. https://doi.org/10.3389/fpsyt.2025.1596625

Polhemus, A., Simblett, S., Dawe-Lane, E., Gilpin, G., Elliott, B., Jilka, S., Novak, J., Nica, R., Temesi, G., & Wykes, T. (2022). Health tracking via mobile apps for depression self-management: A qualitative content analysis of user reviews. *JMIR Human Factors, 9*(4). https://doi.org/10.2196/40133

Pollock, D. M. (2024, September 9). *How to appeal Wegovy insurance coverage denial*. Medical News Today. https://www.medicalnewstoday.com/articles/drugs-how-to-appeal-wegovy-denial

Prasad-Reddy, L., & Isaacs, D. (2015). A clinical review of GLP-1 receptor agonists: efficacy and safety in diabetes and beyond. *Drugs in Context, 4*(212283). https://doi.org/10.7573/dic.212283

Puddick, R. (2025, August 28). *Do you lose more weight on the higher doses of Mounjaro?* Second Nature. https://www.secondnature.io/guides/weight-loss-medications/higher-doses-of-mounjaro?srsltid=AfmBOora89TepMSEfo2mRLiMMgAl0t-kGMXXruzPa_WDxYiLFp2oHxMy

Pursey, K. M., Stanwell, P., Callister, R. J., Brain, K., Collins, C. E., & Burrows, T. L. (2014). Neural responses to visual food cues according to weight status: A systematic review of functional magnetic resonance imaging studies. *Frontiers in Nutrition, 1*. https://doi.org/10.3389/fnut.2014.00007

Reynolds, J. (2025, May 14). *Lotus weight loss clinic.* Lotus Weight Loss. https://lotusweightloss.co.uk/what-are-the-most-common-side-effects-of-mounjaro-vs-wegovy/

Riddle, M. C., Gerstein, H. C., Holman, R. R., Inzucchi, S. E., Zinman, B., Zoungas, S., & Cefalu, W. T. (2018). A1C targets should be personalized to maximize benefits while limiting risks. *Diabetes Care*, *41*(6), 1121–1124. https://doi.org/10.2337/dci18-0018

Rosenbaum, M., & Leibel, R. L. (2010). Adaptive thermogenesis in humans. *International Journal of Obesity*, *34*(S1), S47–S55. https://doi.org/10.1038/ijo.2010.184

Rybelsus dosage guide. (2024, December 9). Drugs.com. https://www.drugs.com/dosage/rybelsus.html

Schnabel, J. (2025, September 23). *Oral GLP-1 drug promotes substantial weight loss in trial.* Cornell Chronicle. https://news.cornell.edu/stories/2025/09/oral-glp-1-drug-promotes-substantial-weight-loss-trial

Semaglutide (oral route). (n.d.). Mayo Clinic. https://www.mayoclinic.org/drugs-supplements/semaglutide-oral-route/description/drg-20492085

Shyam, S., Lee, K. X., Tan, A. S. W., Khoo, T. A., Harikrishnan, S., Lalani, S. A., & Ramadas, A. (2022). Effect of personalized nutrition on dietary, physical activity, and health outcomes: A systematic review of randomized trials. *Nutrients*, *14*(19), 4104. https://doi.org/10.3390/nu14194104

Šoková, B., Greškovičová, K., Halamová, J., & Baránková, M. (2025). Breaking the vicious cycles of self-criticism: a qualitative study on the best practices of overcoming one's inner critic. *BMC Psychology*, *13*(1). https://doi.org/10.1186/s40359-024-02250-2

Stanford, J. (2025, June 26). *Ozempic vs Wegovy: Important differences to consider.* Drugwatch.com. https://www.drugwatch.com/drugs/ozempic/wegovy/

Strumila, R., Lengvenyte, A., Guillaume, S., Nobile, B., Olie, E., & Courtet, P. (2024). GLP-1 agonists and risk of suicidal thoughts and behaviours: Confound by indication once again? A narrative review. *European Neuropsychopharmacology*, *87*, 29–34. https://doi.org/10.1016/j.euroneuro.2024.07.001

Sustainability Directory. (2025, April 28). *Behavioral drift.* https://lifestyle.sustainability-directory.com/term/behavioral-drift/

Tahreem, A., Rakha, A., Rabail, R., Nazir, A., Socol, C. T., Maerescu, C. M., & Aadil, R. M. (2022). Fad diets: Facts and fiction. *Frontiers in Nutrition*, *9*(9). National Library of Medicine. https://doi.org/10.3389/fnut.2022.960922

Turabi, A. E, Ungerman, D., Ahlawat, H, & Hartenstein, L. (2025, May 20). *The path toward a metabolic health revolution.* McKinsey & Company. https://www.mckinsey.com/mhi/our-insights/the-path-toward-a-metabolic-health-revolution

Varajão, J., Magalhães, L., Freitas, L., & Rocha, P. (2022). Success management – From theory to practice. *International Journal of Project Management*, *40*(5). https://doi.org/10.1016/j.ijproman.2022.04.002

Villaines, Z. (2025, April 10). *Headache, nausea, dizziness, fatigue, and stomach pain: Cause.* Medical News Today. https://www.medicalnewstoday.com/articles/headache-nausea-dizziness-fatigue-abdominal-pain

Wong, M. Y. C., Fung, H. W., Wong, J. Y.-H., & Lam, S. K. K. (2025). Exploring the longitudinal dynamics of self-criticism, self-compassion, psychological flexibility, and mental health in a three-wave study. *Scientific Reports*, *15*(1). https://doi.org/10.1038/s41598-025-95821-1

Xing, J. H., & Soffer, E. E. (2001). Adverse effects of laxatives. *Diseases of the Colon and Rectum*, *44*(8), 1201–1209. https://doi.org/10.1007/bf02234645

Zambon, V. (2020, March 26). *Headache, nausea, and fatigue: How are they related?* Medical News Today. https://www.medicalnewstoday.com/articles/headache-nausea-fatigue

Printed in Dunstable, United Kingdom

83208228R00117